LACRYMA CHRISTI

Bernie Unrau DDS

Caltex Press

Published by CalteX Press
3413 16320 24 St SW
Calgary AB T2Y5A1
403-246-0523
www.caltexpress.com

 This novel is a work of fiction. Names, descriptions, entities and incidents included in the story are products of the author's imagination. Any resemblance to actual persons, events and entities is entirely coincidental.

ISBN 978-09866245-6-8

Printed by Amazon in San Bernardino, CA, US; Monee, IL, US; Fort Worth, TX, US; Philadelphia, PA, US; Columbia, SC, US; Mississauga, Ontario, CA; Leipzig, DE, EU; Luton, UK, EU; Torino, IT, EU; Narita, Chiba, JP; Wrocław, Poland, EU
https://www.amazon.com/-/e/B081M9Y1J9

Lacryma Christi c2015

1) Sea Cruise
2) Casablanca
3) Cape of Good Hope
4) Bright Eyes
5) If
6) Pino(t)cchio
7) On The Rocks
8) Eye in the Sky
9) The Eyes Have It
10) Land’s End
11) Providence

PROLOGUE

Ebola, that dreaded, deadly resilient virus that seems to linger, oft for decades in an unsuspecting host only to return with a vengeance. In this case, discovered in the victim's eye. Cloaked either in cartilage due to its poor vascular supply, the eye-ball or semen, endowed with inherent 'immune privileges', the evasive entity resurfaced with a vengeance in a victim deemed medically fit after a fierce bought with the feisty fiend. A medical hero who fought valiantly on the front lines miraculous-ly survived a recurring, never ending battle with the tiny "beast". A potential bioweapon? Another cold war waiting to occur? Various contagions locked away in secret military installations' vaults? One shudders at the thought. It does raise a conten-tious issue and lingering question, are we truly pro-tected from a global pandemic?

Will broke down as he knelt before the deceased woman. Always willing and able to tackle the toughest assignment, Will shuddered as he peered into the bloody eye sockets of the victim. Her delicate high cheekbone structure and ever so slightly curved lips reminded him of his ….fiance.

He slowly, defiantly removed his mask and leaned into the female. The image was indelibly etched in his mind's eye. He jerked back and caught the corner of his suit on a protruding bone, the result of a compound fracture. He felt the sharp edges pen-etrate the fabric, then his own flesh and blood.

"You OK?"

Will froze, arose and arched his aching back. His weary bones the worse for wear.

The chief medical officer noticed the fear that enveloped Will.

"Reminds me of Emma."

"Don't dwell on it. It'll eat you alive."

"Thank God she's a million miles from this hell hole."

"Cheer up, you'll be together soon."

There was little relief in the statement due to its ominous prophetic potential.

"You're vacay begins in less than a week. Where you headed?"

"Casablanca."

"'Heaven Can Wait' assured the commanding officer as he alluded to the original score from the film. "But we can't, come on." The seasoned medical officer spotted the torn fabric of Will's hazmat suit as he turned his attention to the overwhelming task.

"Better let me have a look at that."

"Only a scratch."

The eagle eyes examined the laceration with a degree of concern. He attentively dressed it.

"You've been exposed. I'll have to quarantine you."

" Just what the doctor ordered, huh?"

"You're one of the lucky ones…this stuff's worth it's weight in gold and back ordered for months.

He removed a vial of a potent experimental vaccine produced presumably by Mapp Biopharmaceuticals and a number of new start up firms, then quickly injected the ZMapp concoction into the upper posterior gluteus maximus of the patient.

"Oww. Can't a guy get a break?"

"This is no picnic son. You know what we're up against."

The sweltering heat relented as the sun slipped below the hills. Fifty shades of pale grey filtered through the palm fronds then transformed into a pitch black. A soothing silence descended upon the decimated village, one found in a funeral home.

"Let's light 'em up."

The flame throwers lit up the night sky like tiki torches at a Hawaiian luau. Several of the medics dreamt of roast boar, apples stuffed in their mouths over a steaming spit as tropical maidens' hips swayed to a soothing enchanting beat. Their thirst quenched by an intoxicating elixir. It served as a powerful placebo to mask the gruesome reality that was and could've conceivably spread like a brush fire to consume much of humanity.

The medical party packed up their gear….and left

the smoldering embers..... like happy campers embarking on a desperately sought escape into the back country.

The Huey helicopters whisked the team high above the battlefield like the days of the Vietnam, Korean, Afghanistan or ISIS wars. This was a fight they couldn't lose. A wretched reminder of how susceptible mankind was to such a tiny elusive virulent invader that reared its ugly head regularly to feast on the unsuspecting hosts like rabid vampires or vultures. The formation veered due south over the dense foliage of the rain forest.

"Good riddance. If I ever come this way again, It'll be too soon."

Will was giddy with anticipation. Coupled with sheer fatigue and the warm fuzzy feeling that enveloped him, the result of the vaccine he reasoned.

Will peered into the mirror of the infirmary, situated near the center of the base in Cape Town then straightened his tie and brushed his lapels. He examined his face, studying each aging line that enveloped it. Wrinkles of wisdom he called them. Luckily, he had responded well to the vaccine.

"By the grace of God… Thank you."

"All gussied up for your gal?"

"You've been given a clean bill of health you lucky dog."

Will turned his Mercedes 230 Kompressor off the old main road into the exclusive gated community of Croydon Estates SE of Cape Town. He parked the vehicle, unloaded his gear then approached his fiancee's fashionable custom designed Steenkamp Manor home.

Emma rushed to the door in a bright airy floral print dress with baited breath.

"Honey, I'm home" announced her eager suitor. He dropped his resilient backpacks and stretched out his arms. The two collided in a passionate embrace like sub atomic particles.

Emma was in tears.

"I've been waiting. Fourteen days, 6 hours and 37 minutes to be exact." She smothered him in kisses.

"Let me have a look at you" she begged prying herself from his relentless grip.

"Not so fast" he insisted as he spun her around and reached up to cover her eyes. "No peeking. Promise."

"I promise."

He reached down and unzipped one of the small compartments on his weather beaten backpack then produced a pair of tickets. “Stick out your hands.”

“I love surprises” she cooed.

He placed them tenderly into her sweaty palms.

“I can’t wait.”

“OK, open them. Two tickets to paradise.”

A smile erupted and stretched across her face as she read the words “Aqua Dream” and Morocco Mall….visions of fanciful spending sprees danced in her head.

“Casablanca to be precise.”

“I love you so much.” She assumed two first class air fare tickets to spend as many hours with her honey. Emma placed her sunburnt white bony hands on the cheeks of her dark skinned suitor.

“Did you lose one?”

He was at a loss.

"When did you start wearing contacts?"

"You know I don't wear contacts."

He rushed across to the large vanity mirror in the foyer. Will was astonished by the latest development. He noticed two distinct colors in each eye. One hazel, one dark brown. Artifact? Side effect of the ebola vaccine? A few assorted reports had claimed that ebola could reside in the eyeball and change the pigment of the iris. Will raced into the adjoining bathroom and flushed his eyes feverishly. A puzzled dark complexion stared back at him from the elegant gold rimmed mirror. For a moment Will thought he caught a glimpse of a pale ghostly doppelganger for an instant, double vision? Another side effect of the vaccine? Will reassured himself he was given a clean bill of health. Mission accomplished. The preliminary CDC and WHO updates confirmed that the outbreak had been contained and confined to Liberia, Sierre Leone and Guinea. Will breathed a sigh of relief then turned his attention to the apple of his eye. He knew their children would be smart and beautiful.

After a lengthy lusty, lovemaking interlude the couple came back to their senses, energized, ready to embark on their African extravaganza.

"The skyline hasn't changed a bit."

"You've only been gone two weeks, silly."

"Except for that new 16 story condo complex in the middle of the port."

The yellow cab veered onto the main dock district. The massive mobile oblong structure, the length of 3 football fields, so out of place, housed some 6660 passengers and 2400 crew, dwarfed everything around it.

"Bon Voyage. Cheerio." The cabbie hurriedly unloaded their baggage, raced off, hoping to snatch a few more fares.

"Welcome aboard 'Mystique of the Seas', she's a floating fantasy, a veritable Vegas Resort" stated the seasoned cruise line captain as he extended a hand.

"What happens on board, stays on board, huh?" There was a pause and silence. Will extended his hand. "Will Chambers and this is my fiancée Emma Wilson."

"We're going to get married in Casablanca" she stated anxiously.

"Such a lovely couple, check out Central Park. We have a big surprise in store for our newlyweds and soon to be brides and grooms. "

"I can't wait."

The couple made their way through the maze of decks and myriad of mesmerized passengers to a vantage point in “Central Park”, a 5 story garden atrium lined with fancy boutiques, gift shops, restaurants, even a carousel. It split two sets of swanky state rooms and passenger suites situated along either periphery of the tropical park. Toward the bow a waterslide wove its way around the top deck like a giant anaconda serpent.

The couple sought serenity and refuge in the solarium amongst several like minded wayfarers. The tranquil pool and reclining loungers allowed Will and Emma to reenergize in preparation of the evening festivities. They wiled away the afternoon oblivious of time and space. Only the gentle rocking motion of the massive marine marvel gave away any indication they were still earthbound. Emma’s loss of elapsed time resulted in a rather severe rock lobster red sunburn while Will's kinks and bruises bore the brunt of the intense African sun. Nothing the exclusive spa couldn't work out.

A gala dinner ensued. Several venues to choose from delighted the guests, young and old alike.

"Let's razzle dazzle 'em" stated Emma from the ensuite of their spacious Royal Loft Suite as she affixed her diamond earrings delicately to each lobe. She brushed her fingers through her long blond strands. Something was missing she mulled. A necklace? Emma examined her long ring finger. A piece of the puzzle that may yet be found during the scheduled stop at the site of the former dia-mond rush at Luderitz. It might be just what the doctor ordered as she stepped out of the master suite. The decadent décor coupled with the choice of upstairs / downstairs boudoirs gave them a variety of Vegas like options. The massive dining and living area faced a two story wall to wall ocean view onto a private deck complete with a hot tub and hanging swing basket for two.

"Whatever baby wants, baby gets" insisted Will wantonly as he wrapped his arms around his fiery blonde haired fiancée. They slowly sauntered from their elegant abode down the glass elevator through Central Park to the dazzling club overlooking the Boardwalk below. Countless guests savored the sweet nectar of the gods, select wines from spon-sored vintners, tempting cocktails and treats and to top it off, a Marilyn Monroe impersonator. They spotted their "reserved" table and bolted for the dance floor as a chorus of "Diamonds are a
Girl's Best Friend" began.

The French are glad to die for love.

They delight in fighting duels

But I prefer a man who lives

And gives expensive jewels.

A kiss on the hand

May be quite continental,

But diamonds are a girl's best friend.

A suave Michael Buble look alike sauntered on the stage hoping to woo his high maintenance gal.

A kiss may be grand

But it won't pay the rental

On your humble flat

Or help you at the automat.

Men grow cold

As girls grow old,

And we all lose our charms in the end.

But square-cut or pear-shaped,

These rocks don't lose their shape.

Diamonds are a girl's best friend…

Michael countered with "As Time Goes By" to try to win the affection of his woman. The timeless masterpiece from the film "Casablanca" stirred the crowd noticeably.

You must remember this
A kiss is just a kiss,
a sigh is just a sigh
the fundamental things apply
as time goes by
And when two lovers woo
They still say I love you....

Emma mimicked the words in sync with Will... The spotlight illuminated the couple, completely immersed in each other's arms.

On that you can rely
No matter what the future brings...
As time goes by
Moonlight and love songs

Never out of date

Hearts full of passion

Jealousy and hate

Woman needs man

And man must have his mate….

A slightly sloshed man resembling Eric the Red stumbled toward the dance floor…disturbed by the display….

That no one can deny

It's still the same old story

A fight for love and glory….

Michael Buble's double noticed the inebriated patron push a few dancers aside. He clearly had his eye on Emma.

"Let's pick up the pace…a little" as he motioned for security to step in. "Here's an all time favorite:

I took my baby

On a Saturday bang

Boy is that girl with you

Yes we're one and the same

Now I believe in miracles

And a miracle has happened tonight

But if you're thinkin' bout my baby

Doesn't matter if you're black or white

"Of all the gin joints onboard, she walks into mine." The fiery 'Eric the Red' stormed onto the stage in a rage of fury….either infatuated with a female sporting the the same sunburnt complexion or extremely perturbed by the interracial antics. No one knew before it was too late.

"Excuse me, mind if I dance?" he asked Emma pushing Will aside.

"Hey buddy, she's with me" defended Will.

"I didn't ashhhk you" slurred the tipsy bleary eyed tourist. He grabbed Emma firmly around the waist and pulled her toward him. Will could not stand idly by. He pushed the drunk away. In response the man clenched his fists and replied:

"Don't you see it matters? Everything matters." He wound up with a wicked left hook. It caught Will in the left cheekbone, deflected up into his left orbit. The force of the impact ruptured and crushed his eyeball, in fact dislodged his retina. The ebola virus laced spray of blood shot across the dance floor. It caught the captain in the face as he was about to give his welcome speech. It doused a waiter, a few patrons and security guards that quickly tackled the drunk. It severely marred the momentum of an otherwise memorable evening.

Will dropped to the floor TKO. His jaw hit the deck hard. The virus tainted blood in his eye shot through his venous return system directly to his brain. In the ensuing confusion, the waiter brushed his blood stained uniform, that further spread the infectious virus laden aerosolized blood to a number of adjacent tables and horrified guests who panicked and tried to shake it off further dissipating the dreaded disease. The captain rushed to the front of the stage and grabbed the mike from Michael.

"Ladies and gentlemen, please remain calm."

"Looks like we might have a mutiny on our hands" quipped a sloshed guest.

"Please, I assure you it's simply a little mis-understanding" pleaded the captain eager to save face and the potential of frivolous lawsuits against the cruise lines. The feisty redheaded Irishman refused to go quietly into the night. He struggled and squirmed then sneezed violently onto several guests. They were appalled and left in disgust. The virus had now found several unsuspecting hosts from which to stage an elusive advance. Soon free to roam the world's largest ocean liner and wreak absolute havoc.

"He must be allergic to love" quipped an audience member. "All's fair in love and war" added another inebriated patron.

Michael picked up the tempo, where he had left off undeterred by the "heckler".

I am tired of this devil
I am tired of this stuff
I am tired of this business
So when the going gets rough
I ain't scared of your brother
I ain't scared of no sheets....

The ship staff quickly removed the stained white table cloths... further exposing themselves to the virus. The sheets were quickly carried to the laundry where several passengers brushed against the tainted blood stained sheets. More handlers were exposed to the tablecloths as housekeeping curiously examined the stain, feverishly rubbing it before immersing it in a blood bath. The waiter contaminated the plates as he carried them to the kitchen from each table. The kitchen staff wiped the bloody tainted food into the sink. A dishwasher broke a glass in the confusion and allowed the virus to enter the open wound unawares. Ebola now had the run of the ship, exposing several vital services onboard.

Emma rushed to Will's side where a few guests gently rolled him onto his back. Before the ship's physician arrived several snake oil salesmen aka amateur medics touched the tender cheek bone exposing themselves .to the virus released from the confines of the immunologically 'privileged' orbit of Will's left eyeball.

"Please. That's quite alright, he's a doctor" insisted Emma as she pushed the well wishing patrons aside to let Will catch his breath.

A smile broke out across his bloody face as he forced his right eye open and caught a glimpse of his true love. The apple of his eye. He'd die for her. Proof was in the pudding. The ship's captain accompanied by several EMS quickly hoisted Will onto a stretcher.

"I'm OK, I think I can walk" he stated confidently albeit woozy. He toppled like a drunken sailor…landing on another unsuspecting couple. The world's deadliest virus waiting for the perfect moment, unleashed, by a comedy of errors, the inception set into motion a series of irreversible events .

"All the world's a stage, All the men and

women merely players, they have their exits and entrances, and one man in his time plays many parts" stated Will ominously, eerily prophetically quoting Shakespeare's "As You Like It", 7 ages of man from birth to inevitable, imminent miserable death. Will tried to focus and mull over the mean-ing only for a moment in his concussed state.

"Are you sure you're alright?"

"I'll be fine" insisted the seasoned military physician and virologist.

"Nothin' doin'. Air Mercy Service? We're going to need an AW 119 STAT....air lift you to Cape Town. Let an ophthalmologist have a look at you. We'll also need x-rays for a possible cheek bone fracture and an avulsed left eye" said the ship's physician. "You took quite a left hook lad."

The AMS AW 119 Koala responded instantly...

Within minutes they were airborne.

"They can pick up the patient from the basket-ball court up top."

"Roger that."

Several spotlights lit up the night sky like a Hollywood premiere. She stood out like a sore thumb on the pitch black south Atlantic.

"There she is" noted the copilot. Most of the porch lights muted the main beam rising from mid ship like a laser beam.

"We'll set her down up top, there."

"Roger that."

The patient's gurney was wheeled across center court and whisked aboard his waiting chariot.

"You took quite a left hook lad" stated the EMS flight surgeon as he examined Will's lacerated face. He probed the bloody eye socket to determine the extent of the injury then shook his head. The nurse cringed. She applied a banana bag drip and attached several leads and took Will's vital signs. "You're lucky to be alive."

"Yeah, it's my lucky day."

The nurse wiped the wound clean while the doc meticulously wrapped a dressing around Will's head. The dabbed cotton dropped to the floor of the chopper.

"Where you from?"

"Cape Town."

"Allergic to anything?"

"No." The nurse stuck an ampicillin filled syringe into his arm.

"Ever been sick in hospital?"

She flipped through the lengthy medical history questionnaire…awaiting an answer. She fidgeted with her pen, clicking it repeatedly. Time was of the essence.

“Uh actually....” Will paused. Not wanting to alarm anyone by revealing the fact he had been exposed to the Ebola virus in Guinea. Treated. Given a clean bill of health. No point spreading pandemonium throughout the vessel. A confined space. Close quarters. Sharing the same water, food. Over 9000 potential victims, 6660 passeng-ers, 2400 crew at the mercy of one highly danger-ous escapee ...the Ebola virus. He was torn. How bad could it get? Will wasn’t thinking straight in his concussed state coupled with the incipient onset of symptoms of hemorrhagic fever.

“No.”

The AW 119 KE approached the port district. The large landmark, Cape Town Stadium, like an ever present eye followed the descent just to the east in a grassy area near New Somerset Hospital.

The virus had gained its first port of entry as the patient was wheeled inside the emergency section. Will's head spun bordering on an epileptic seizure as he watched the rows of lights flash by overhead.

"You're gonna be alright son" stated the confident voice of the chief surgical resident. "Let's take a few pictures" as they sat him upright in the panoramic, cephalogram x-ray and MRI units.

"That's my good side" quipped Will.

"Smile."

The images revealed a slight cheek bone fracture but the damage had been done. Inspite of the best efforts to control the swelling, the virus had spread to the brain, bathing its vital processes like an effervescent fountain. The cells divided extremely rapidly. It was only a matter of days before the first signs of bleeding around the eye erupted, in time every orifice occurred. Then as the virus literally tore all the cellular membranes apart in each organ system in its insidious inva-sion, Will would be reduced to a bloody mushy mess. The words Clean Bill of Health popped onto the large flat screen as the staff pulled his medical records.

"Well I'll be a monkey's uncle" said the surgical resident astonished. "Chief virologist MSF Medecins Sans Frontieres, Doctors Without Bor-ders. Recent stints in Guinea and Liberia to combat ebola." As he turned to the nurse, she cringed.

"Out of the frying pan…"

--

The savory aroma permeated the fully equipped culinary laboratory as the flames danced higher. The connoisseurs busily sprinkled the garnishes and added the finishing touches to an endless array of filet mignons, New York strip, rib eye, T-bone, seared, braised, grilled to perfection.

Emma summoned all her strength and reluctantly joined a small group of single women on girl's night out at the Chop Grille on the Promenade deck. First a short pit stop at Vintages. Rather than stew over the unfortunate turn of events in her spacious Royal Loft Suite alone, and watch endless reruns of Casablanca, the sound of another human with the remote possibility of a consoling con-versation lifted her spirits. An eternal optimist, she knew her husband was a fighter, not in the traditional ring, but when facing an elusive foe or challenging medical puzzle he was at his best. He'd come back from the gates of hell before. In a matter of days he'd join her and walk her down the aisle in holy matrimony to begin the rest of their lives together. Come what may. She raised her glass of finc wine:

"To love."

"To love" echoed the cackle of curvaceous chicks.

"Here's to all the lying, stealing, cheating drunks of the world" said a saucy spinster.

"I've never cheated on Will….why I…"

"If you must lie, lie in the arms of the one you love, and if you're gonna steal, steal their heart too, if you must cheat, cheat death and if you drink, drink to…

"Me, drink to my health, you know I can't drink anymore" interjected the loud lush with the immortal last words of Picasso by McCartney & Wings.

"No, drink to the moments that take your breath away" explained the intoxicated enchantress examining her empty life. She'd buried her fourth husband. Number five was waiting just around the corner, she assured herself. Perhaps she'd pick up something or someone at the exclusive DeBeers gift shop.

Several notices were sent to each passenger's state room, even their personal ipad or smart phone

informing them of a slight change in plans. Not a significant detour per se, but in light of the Ebola scare in several African countries inland excursions or scheduled stops were reduced to a select few. Just to be safe? Rather hypocritical. The fatal fax pas had been overlooked entirely. The first commandment of a physician's lengthy curriculum, the Hippocratic Oath – "Do No Harm". And he of all people had been whisked to safety. Oh the irony.

Emma awoke from a sleepless night wrapped in the luxurious silky sheets, the only immediate temporary relief. She had tossed and turned all night. Her leg stretched out across the vast void. She missed the touch and feel of her mate's body. Emma leapt into the soothing steamy shower and let the gentle pulsing action massage her tense shaking form. She stared out to into a restless empty sea through the large circular porthole then came back to her senses. A significant period of time elapsed before she stepped from the safety of her steamy tropical enclosure.

Emma pressed the hot iron into the fabric of the tan safari blouse in preparation of the short 'excursion' scheduled later that morning.

Enroute to the departure deck Emma bumped into the captain.

"I can't thank you enough for all you've done …Captain?"

"Captain Calhoun at your service, Emma is it? Sorry your cruise began on such a sour note. Your fiance'll be fine. I want to assure everyone has a pleasant voyage, and I mean everyone."

"You don't know what that means to me" she smiled. Mind if I…? She held up her smartphone for a quick selfie.

"Not at all, my pleasure."

She snapped a few pics. This sea faring voyage was anything but unforgettable thus far.

"Enjoy your trip."

"Thank you." The captain coughed and suddenly became weak in his knees. So out of character for the salty sea dog. He smiled at her and quickly regained his composure.

"You're not falling for me too are you captain?" quipped Emma. His embarrassed face bore a bright cherry red glow.

A small group of eager explorers gathered at the departure point and climbed aboard the rugged reinforced rubber raft.

The zodiac dashed across the waves toward the edge of the Namibia desert, a dry sandy foreboding wasteland. The tour guide's voice roared above the outboard.

"We'll visit a small abandoned ghost town, Kolman'skop, where the 1st diamond was discover-ed by a worker back in 1908. In fact they were literally found at one's feet all over the place." The group scoured the sandy beach below their sandals as they disembarked, eagerly hoping. Keenly aware of the possibilities that each shiny pebble held.

"Oh by the way we have provided permits for all of you. It set in motion a mecca of mining mavens and magnates. CDM Consolidated diamond mines of SW Africa was established in 1928 by Sir Ernest Oppenheimer. Wealth beyond their wildest dreams. A town soon sprung up including a hospital,
school, even a casino and ballroom and the 1st tram in Africa."

Emma was overcome by the abandoned barren wasteland...completely inundated by wind driven sand dunes. The stark sole survivor was the mine manager's home which seemed unscathed.

"In 1994 CDM and the government of Namibia formed Namdeb." One of the passengers erupted in a violent series of sneezes as she entered. The stale air thought to be the cause... yet the bloody sputum that sprayed the walls of the vacant dwelling alarmed Emma. It evoked images of the bloody sacrifices of the slave workers, many of whom were slaughtered

"My God! You're coming down with one nasty cold." It was then she realized the woman was seated near the dance floor where her husband had been assaulted.

"Project 2050 established back in 2010 set in motion the means to insure fair sustained growth. In 2011 the Namibian government and DeBeers equalized the shareholding structure."

The search party left empty handed eager to sample the fruits of the labors of Namdeb in the exclusive DeBeers gift shop.

Day 4 into the excursion sent shock waves throughout the ship. Many of the delectable diners and irresistible restaurants sat vacant. The usual hustle and bustle of the interactive promenades now echoed the emptiness of a few brave souls footsteps who ventured about the ship. The spirited fitness hosted venues desperately sought participants. The majority of guests were rendered rather incapacitated, either bedridden in their berths and state rooms or the ship's well equipped infirmaries.

It struck every socioeconomic class. No one was immune from the rapid spread of the viral outbreak. The captain and crew were equally stricken. The bridge now a bare bones rag tag team of the most resistant seamen. In the overcrowded infirmary, the ship's physician leafed through the downloaded version of Harrison's Internal Medicine text on his laptop and the iDoc diagnostic app on his smartphone. Even the recent CDC updates reported no new outbreaks of Ebola. He desperately sought an answer to the overwhelming number of cases, all exhibiting the same sym-ptoms. Red eyes, bleeding from orifices in the later stages, chest pain, stomach aches, nausea, vomiting, diarrhea. It took a severe toll on the ship's already overburdened plumbing A few pipes burst spewing the bloody exudate into long vast corridors. It left no stone unturned as it contaminated the cleaning crews.

"It's happening so fast" he said worriedly to his nursing staff and peered around the room. The supply of antibiotics and analgesics was despe-rately low. A sick feeling permeated the pit of his stomach. The likelihood of a full blown out of control epidemic now very much in the realm of possibility. Barred from any port of entry. But he wouldn't be the harbinger of bad news and dampen their spirits. He'd pass the buck on to the captain. Ultimately the fate of each passenger rested in his capable hands. He smiled at the noticeably pertur-bed nursing staff.

Emma examined the selfie all alone on the large empty balcony. Odd, the captain exhibited the same bizarre hazel/brown ocular anomaly as Will did. Or was it because her loving soul mate was foremost on her mind? Every passenger began to remind her of Will, exhibiting the same similar anomaly. Was she going out of her mind? She got up woozily. The gentle rocking of the vessel began to disturb her. She fished through her purse for a Gravol to combat the motion sickness. In lieu of her usual remedy she found a syringe labelled "just in case" obviously stashed by her fiancé.

Struggling to focus on the tiny print,

"zee…mupp…et", she laughed, envisioning Ernie's embrace in lieu of her fiance's and jabbed her thigh. Emma decided to soak her weary bones and worried mind in a long, luxurious bubble bath., her faithful companion by her side…one rubber duckie.

“Who’s up for a walk on the wild side? Don’t be shy” quipped the tour guide. The joke shot over the heads of the guests strong enough for the outing; those who sought escape inspite of the warnings against disembarking onto African soil. “Shai game reserve offers a brush with nature at it’s most pristine. We’ll see a plethora of Senegal parrots, swallow tailed bee-eaters….and even baboons and monkeys.” They passed by a local casket maker’s shop piqued by the intricately carved images. The life stories and tall tales that had made their lives unique were etched along the sides of each long wooden box. A few tourists paused and shuddered facing their own mortality. A stark reminder of the twist of fate that led to the inevitable ending.

An equally unwelcome sight, noted the seasoned guide, was the swarm of black tipped birds of prey circling high overhead. They followed the landing party every step of the way like predator drones.

"Let's stay close together."

A middle aged couple succumbed to the heat and lost their way. They wandered from the group and soon came within a stone's throw of a few gorillas. Whether the heat, sheer excitement or fear caused them to collapse, was of no concern to the feisty famished beasts. With no hesitation or reservation the menacing gorillas gored and noshed on the bloody victims. Ebola was passed from human host back to gorilla. The macabre circle of life now complete. Ebola was originally thought to be ingested by tribes eating tainted gorilla meat. Hakuna Matata? No worries? Be happy? As the sated simians left the spoils to the next in line, a swarm of black tipped birds of prey swooped in for the fiesta resistance. The deviation from their usual flight path had proven highly profitable indeed.

Emma returned from the invigorating excursion if only to get away from the ghastly ghostly void of the vessel. Reduced to a skeleton crew, nare a porter or shop keeper was to be found. She wondered where all the crew were? Let alone the passengers. Had they expired? Was there a make-shift morgue onboard? She shuddered at the thought. In the ship's infirmary a sheet was drawn over the face of another victim. The blood oozed from each orifice onto the bed. The ship physician drenched in the soaked blood, sweat and tears sat in shock as he peered about the chamber of horrors. A few bright red drops dripped from his nose onto his smartphone. The iDoc app quickly analyzed the blood sample and spewed out the inevitable prognosis, death…by… Ebola virus disease. He shut off the electronic device.

One port of call remained prior to the final destination. The number of partakers had dwindled drastically. Many reached their expiry date far too soon for their maker, soon in the hands of an undertaker. The perplexing marine enigma had taken its toll. Even the ship's physician had succumbed to the virus from early exposures to infected passengers. It had run its fatal course in a matter of 3 days to a week. Why the warning signs were not heeded or reacted upon more seriously we may never know. Was it the captain's decision to avoid pandemonium at sea, perhaps causing a mass mutiny? Or worse the ship banned from reentering any port? Perhaps this was why a small group of resourceful, resilient souls sought to abandon ship, The only recourse under the disguise of a directed tour.

The small Zodiaks clipped across the still waters off the coast of Fuerteventura or "winds of fort-une". Located on the leeward side in the small chain of Canary Islands, it was also the most isolated. The eager explorers anxiously waited to set foot on the seldom visited shores of the UN-ESCO world biosphere reserve like the mission-aries did so many years ago on some distant tropical isle or as Neil Armstrong once ventured on the moon. They touched down on the black sands of 'Caleta Negrae' meaning black bay in

Spanish. They sought relief any way they could to escape from the congested, death ridden belly of the beast as Jonah once sought to flee from his hellish afflic-tion. The crazed infected few who remained alive kissed the ground as if it were sacred. They'd spend the last few hours of their lives in paradise.

The consolation prize, a bitter pill to swallow.

A few bleary bloody eyed survivors scoured the small beach then sought to search inland for an ounce of hope. A noted ornithologist spotted the unique black wing tips of the birds of prey overhead.

"Ayy, they've been waiting" he coughed be-tween sentences. He'd soon succumb to the scourge that had spread through the ship like the plague or a brush fire. "Wretched Egyptian vul-tures, Pharoah's chicken. Revered by ISIS, the goddess of wisdom, marriage and health, ha!" He coughed up a bloody sputum and sprayed the beach. The onlookers ogled, they knew they'd soon be next. "According to the Greek legend, Aegyp-ius the friend of Nephreon was having an affair with his mother Timandra. Nephreon sought revenge. He sowed the seeds of his own destruct-ion by tricking Bulis, Aegypius' mother to sleep with her son in a darkened chamber."

"Ohh my…" sighed the spectators.

"Bulis was so disgusted she scratched out his eyes before killing herself. Aegypius prayed for revenge. Zeus meted out a chilling punishment by…turning them both into vultures forever preying on the….." the tour guide didn't even complete his short story ere he expired.

The sparsely populated island save for but a few locals and indigenous flora and fauna seemed the ideal place to die.

A weary senior had lost the wanderlust. He had lived a good life. His wife now by his side savored the fleeting memories of their golden years and awaited what fate had in store. They kissed each other on the lips as they had thousands of times and cherished the peaceful final chapter of their long well spent lives. They knew they'd be going to a better place in the hereafter. They succumbed shortly thereafter to the effects of the Ebola virus.

A few black winged tipped vultures circled overhead scouring the generous spoils dotting the perimeter of the black bay. The character – istic tips of the predominantly white bird with a golden brownish head, the result of feasting on feces whenever the opportunity arose. They swooped down in a death spiral landing with aerial acrobatic precision and proceeded to pick the tasty Ebola tainted carcasses clean. To the bone. Their sated bellies filled with the harbinger of death. The potential of a global airborne pandemic worse than the Black Plague now hung in the balance. The winds of fate would fling them far and wide in their vast migratory swath stretching across the Mediterranean to Asia minor as far as the eastern tip of India. Soaring on thermals high above at times 500 km /day ISIS's chosen deposited their deadly cargo of eggs embedded with the Ebola virus onto rooftops, cliffs and cavern's cracks. As far north as the black covered lava laden slopes of Mt. Vesuvius. Buried in the sands of the Sahara. In the holiest of holies in Jerusalem. Far beyond the middle east to the Eagle temples of Eastern India in Tamil Nadu.

There the unsuspecting priests inadvertently fed the birds a noon day snack of rice, wheat, sugar and ghee. The birds waited with baited breath to unleash their frenzied wrath upon a billion oblivious Indian inhabitants and seal the fate of countless Hindu worshippers…bird to bird, bird to human, and eventually human to human transmission insured.

The captain struggled, bracing himself against the control console, clearly on his last legs. He peered out into the vast void as he had a thousand times. The ancient mariner found a glimmer of hope. Above the bow of the boat he imagined a flock of albatross to guide them home. The harbinger of good luck was in actuality a swarm of blood thirsty birds of prey. Pharoah's Chicken, the Canary Isle Egyptian Vulture, ISIS' chosen, the grim reapers waiting patiently for a veritable endless smorgasbord about to be offered, to mete out their form of vengeance.

The last man standing. Once full of life, vim and vigor, now a gloomy ghost ship, his crew lay prostrate in pools of their own blood. A similar gory scene was evident on the aqua deck where countless corpses lined the loungers, the sport pool, even the kid's aquatic playground. The exclusive suites staterooms once full of vim and vigor now strewn with bloody corpses stained in their virus ridden vomitus and blood. He corrected the course of the massive marine morgue for the last time. Now a monstrous 'morgue ship' speeding toward it's final destination. The three 16 cylinder Wartsila rail engines still cranked out some 18,860 watts, over 25,000 horses racing toward the finish line at 22.6 knots. He aligned the vessel's com-puter's bearings with a neon emblazoned sign, 'Rick's American Café' nestled near the end of the large port awaiting the Mystique of the Seas. One small detail nagged him. Even the encyclopedic naval knowledge jostling inside his cranium could not come up with a solution. He had navigated many a stormy sea and deep water port, Casa-blanca amongst them in his long illustrious un-blemished naval career. Yet the unfathomable inevitable concern was, how to make a hairpin turn around the lengthy break water wall lining the outskirts to reenter the port. With his dying breath he prayed for forgiveness.

The marine behemoth bore down on the Mor-occo coastline like a crazed convoy of Berbers did so many years ago. An assortment of lights twinkled along the 16 putrid decks of death.

In the distance a spectacular sister ship, the Pride of the Seas, had just left port bound for the Canary Islands on its lengthy leisurely European Cruise.

She'd made the harrowing hairpin turn with the greatest of ease heading westward along the break water wall. An atmosphere of anticipation stirred in the hearts of some 6660 adventurers. Coupled with the generous crew catering to their every heart's desire, the champagne overflowed the fancy Swarovski crystal flutes to the brim. Destined to experience the ultimate in naval extravaganzas, not a care in the world, their worries and woes left onshore. They forgot about time and place as they partied merrily on into the night.

"Here's to the first day of the rest of our lives"

toasted the aging retired honeymooning couple in their finest tuxedo and ball room gown. They intertwined their arms like two intoxicated love birds then downed the bubbly elixir. It tingled in their noses. They tossed the flutes overboard. Out of the corner of their eyes they noted the large towering twinkling tree of lights. It reminded them of Rockefeller Square's finest, much larger coming ever closer.

"WTF?" whaled the wide eyed woozy wayfarer and a handful of equally mystified watchful eyes from their cozy sea side balconies. The disbelief in their eyes of equal magnitude to that fateful morn in 1912 when the ship deemed unsinkable struck a seemingly small, harmless chunk of ice.

Most of the crew and passengers were immersed in the merriment and enticing offerings of Neptune. The finest mahi mahi, salmon, sturgeon, roe, row upon row filled the irresistible reservoirs of decadent delights.

No one could've imagined nor even noticed the imminent event about to change the course of history…forever. Deemed impossible or so remote one would more likely be struck by lightning aboard the vessel twice. Like two subatomic particles in a perfect bull's eye forced upon one another. The end result was an unexpected impact of epic proportions. Ere the captain could even respond, via instant electronic command, the mighty marine engines roared defiantly in a full 360 degree swivel capability, but it was too late. The massive floating hotels merged. Unlike a Trump-Wynn-win deal, the cataclysmic event, like an enormous end of times earthquake rocking Vegas or the free world, tore the Pride of the Seas in two. Blindsided by the Mystique of the Seas, the two largest ships on the high seas today, on a date with destiny, joined in the holiest of shot gun matrimonies and sealed their fates.

The horrendous grating, grinding sound of metal ,deck upon deck. The blunt force tore the façade like a wrapper ripped off a candy bar or tuna can. It sliced the ship in two like an ice pick through butter. Gut wrenching, blood curdling screams echoed from the gaping hole. Like cracked chest-nuts roasting on an open fire, the fiery hellish inferno, now a vast surreal nightmare. Bodies dangled from countless cavernous exposed decks. Many dropped like flies to their doom in the fiery inferno. 18 lifeboats sat on the outside of the shattered vessel along the port and starboard sides sat idly by, unreachable. The bow of the Mystique crumpled and left her innards exposed. Water surged into her massive bloody void like a raging tidewater following a tsunami. Neither the air tight compartment doors, now rendered inoperative, nor the grace of God could conceivably save any of their wretched lives.

Countless rotting Ebola ridden corpses fell from the Mystique of the Seas or were swallowed up in an instant by the Atlantic. Most sought relief by praying for a quick end to the hellish ordeal.

A chaplain fell from his pulpit during an evening service as the Pride of the Seas split in two. The only words he mustered in the midst of the maritime apocalypse, from Revelation 16, verse 3 King James Version of the bible.

"And the second angel poured out his vial upon the sea; and it became as the blood of a dead man; and every living soul died in the sea." His words were drowned out by the screams and pleas amidst the pandemonium. It was the last supper for many.

The massive burial at sea sent shock waves through the water all along the Morocco coastline. The swirling blood bath lured as many as 50 species of sharks from near and far, as far as the Balearic Isles off Spain. Come to sample the spectacular sizeable smorgasbord. It created a feeding frenzy of epic proportions. Great White, Blue, Black Tip, Sand Tiger, even whale sharks. The elusive predator had survived slaughter, pollution, disease and famine for millions of years. Today was a day of reckoning. Payback. Their gaping orifices, lined by razor sharp edges row upon row bore down on the dead or live alike. They did not discriminate. Nor did the Ebola virus. They were equal opportunistic predators Ebola happily took refuge inside it's idyllic new home.

Its host, a highly mobile menacing eating machine bound for the warm sun drenched shores of the southern Mediterranean.

Emma thrashed about in the bloody salty stew strewn with flotsam and jetsam. She was startled merely by the fact of being alive. Several bodies bobbled up and down all around her for a few minutes before they disappeared below the surface. Some dead, some about to drown, many snatched by the gaping hungry jaws of death. The vicious cycle continued for hours ere the search and rescue boats from the port of Casablanca arrived in droves. They approached the scene of the monstrous marine disaster in utter shock and disbelief. No amount of emergency sea rescue simulation or training could've conceivably prepared them for this. After the initial shock, vomiting, screams and utter disbelief subsided, they worked feverishly round the clock. Extracting bodies from the wreckage in an endless ‘red sea’ while fending for themselves from aerial assaults by ISIS’s chosen bird of prey. Many of Pharoah’s chickens were snatched by ecstatic sharks leaping from the water in the feeding frenzy. The spread of the Ebola epidemic was insured, whether by air, land or sea, the vector the ultimate victor in the vicious cycle. Up past the rock of Gibraltar, from the south of Spain , it advanced with a vengeance the world hadn’t seen since the 1918 Spanish Infuenza, which infected half a billion and killed between 50 and 100 million. The Black Death which peaked from 1346-53 killed upwards of 200 million people throughout central Asia and Europe. Both catas-trophies paled in comparison to the magnitude of this emerging menace. Word soon spread like wild fire around the globe. World leaders were on high alert. Plagued with an ever growing immi-gration problem, this catalyst proved to be the straw that broke not only the camel's back in the African nations but European governments as well. Rumors of a shipborne sabotage to ISIS inspired acts of terrorism resonated round the world from the admiral's office, naval headquarters of the US 6th fleet stationed in Naples, Italy to Woods Hole Oceanographic Institute, Massachusetts where the latest research vessel, the RV Neil Armstrong's crew awaited word to set foot on no man's land. It reverberated through the corridors, all the way up the pecking order and food chain to the think tanks quickly assembled outside the oval office in the Whitehouse. The president's finger ever present on the phone, probed and deciphered the endless possibilities of the cause of the calamity. Plans and strategies in place to counter bioterrorist to insidious ISIS led attacks, the joint chiefs of staff edgy, their hair triggers ready to launch a preemptive strike at any second. Immediate emergency medical relief, hazmat teams ever ready to address the hot button issues of the day.

2: Casablanca

> "If that plane leaves the ground and you're not on it, you'll regret it. Maybe not today, maybe not tomorrow, but soon and for the rest of your life."

- Humphrey Bogart, from the 1942 film "Casablanca"

"The perfect storm. I see. They got themselves into one helluva pickle" said the president of the united states perplexed.

"The pickles out of the jar sir, the cat's out of the bag?"

"Let me put it to you this way sir, Pandora's box

has irreversibly, however inadvertently been opened."

"Death and destruction the world has not seen the likes of?" The softly spoken words resonated with everyone in the room. The press secretary quickly prepared a speech for the commander in chief to address the nation and free world. Several joint chiefs of staff mulled their military options. Strike while the iron was hot. Some feared it was already too late for a surprise attack.

"The answer obviously lies at the bottom of Pandora's box…" ruminated the president.

"Oh? You mean the vessel?" the staff, all ears. Their eyes focused on the wrinkled lines of the commander in chief's worried face waiting for his lips to move. They hung on his every word.

"It hasn't eluded us or surfaced yet." They were at a loss. Expecting a magic potion locked in a trunk buried deep within the cargo hold to pop out. "Why hope! Ha, ha" he chuckled nervously.

Finding a survivor amidst the bloody floating debris proved futile for the eagle eyes scouring the sky and aboard the Zodiaks and small vessels which flitted about the flotsam and jetsam. Not a soul surfaced. They were startled. As a last resort, a Marrakech fishing trawler accompanied by a couple of Moroccan warships including the Aquitaine class frigate scoured the perimeter of the Mystique. The crew tossed two large nets over-board and began to harvest a sea of death and destruction.

"Anything?" asked the astonished captain of the Fremm, a modern multi purpose French frigate.

"Slim pickens. Not a soul! They're all dead!" sighed the stunned seaman.

"Sacre bleu."

"Wait!"

"Oui?"

"Good news. A miracle. Word just in, they found a survivor, a young woman near the stern… She said she fell asleep in the Royal Sky Loft Suite. Next thing she found herself adrift in tomato soup, what she thought at first was a bad dream."

"Thank God."

The local fishermen and emergency responders were somewhat luckier scouring the Pride of the Sea's perimeter. The divers, outfitted in hermetic ally sealed neoprene suits, armed with spear guns and all forms of shark repellant fought off the ferocious predators fiercely. Their precious catch of the day, a small percentage of resilient passengers and crew that had survived were pulled from the briny bloody soup.

“The divers found a Samsung smartphone on the bridge, amongst the ravaged bodies and debris, perhaps belonging to the captain. It may give us a clue?”

“Oui. Merci. His state of mind, his last orders” mulled the military marine maven. He radioed the president of Casablanca, Spanish for White House.

“You have our deepest condolences” insisted the Commander.

“5000 Americans aboard the Mystique.”

‘Teach a man to fish, he’ll fish for a lifetime.’

A sick feeling permeated the pit of his stomach. “All hands lost.” The gut wrenching words tightened in the gullet of each officer and joint chief of staff. “Except one young woman…South African …thank you.”

“Only a few fortunate Americans were pulled from the Pride thus far. I see…”

"I want the US 6th fleet to send in a convoy stat."

"On their way, sir" assured retired admiral Jones. "Headed by the USS Mount Whitney", flagship of the fleet, a Blue Ridge Class command ship, the most sophisticated C4i - command, control, communications, computer & intelligence ship ever commissioned. "She'll spearhead a special Task Force, an amphibious attack fleet consisting of one aircraft carrier, USS George H. W. Bush", CVN 77, named after the US Navy's youngest pilot and 41st president. "The USS Ft McHenry" the defense of which inspired the 'Star Spangled Banner', … and received a Meritorious Unit Commendation Award for the Exxon Valdez cleanup. "And a couple of converted San Clemente class supertankers , now fully equipped hospital ships, the USNS Comfort and a 2nd Mercy Class vessel to provide 2000+ hospital beds. An optimistic number I know, in light of the mass mayhem."

"Thank you. I want our brightest and best USAMRIID airborne and onboard the RV Neil Armstrong to investigate STAT."

"The Neil Armstrong?"

"We've set foot on unknown, foreign soil before. Tread where only eagles dare."

"Aye aye sir."

The 238 foot long research vessel lined with the latest virology labs and sophisticated diagnostic equipment to study the surface and subsurface of the oceans lay in its berth. About to embark on a voyage not only out of their comfort zone but area of expertise, the young scientists had no idea what awaited them. Their eager minds had unraveled a few marine enigmas, sources of omega 3 fatty acids formed as a byproduct of a hardy deep sea bacteria and so on.

"Why are they sending us? The only contaminants washing ashore along the pristine Moroccan beaches are the ubiquitous two legged variants. Likely dehydrated or already dead. They'd be better off sending the AFIP" or Armed Forces Institute of Pathology "for mass disaster processing" stated the know it all from behind his coke bottle glasses scouring the laptop screen inundated with data.

"Where have you been, on the moon?" They disestablished that branch in 2011. They moved to Bethesda as the National Medical Marine Center.

"Yeah, so?" snapped the irritated scientist rather lackadaisically.

"Word on the street is a bioterrorist attack…."

"Right up your alley Hatfield". The noted

scientist, not the notorious magician, had fought most of his battles in court rather than the battle-fields or level four containment facilities he had trained at…and won unanimously. Faced with several slanderous, defamatory allegations during the anthrax scares in Virginia, etc he had come out smelling like a rose amongst a bunch of 'thorny pricks', ie the legal beagles who had accused him of masterminding or colluding with colleagues. All hearsay and BS. He defended his name and honor in a fiercely contested legal battle in a court of law. To top it off and spite them even more he named his latest 'hobby' boat, "The Beagle IV" outfitted from the undisclosed multi-million dollar settle-ment from both NSA and government defense departments.

"We'll see" stated the cautious virologist. He chose his words, ways and means more carefully nowadays. Hind sight was always 20-20.

"In any event we can take her for a test drive. This is where the rubber hits the road." He pulled a driver from his golf bag and placed the ball on the makeshift artificial turf. He waited patiently for a military destroyer to pass by lining up his shot.

"Four" he shouted to rub salt into the wounds. The ball bounced off the side of the resilient steel hull with a loud clink and sunk below the surface.

"They've stirred up much more than a hornet's nest."

The CVN-77 approached the Casablanca port authority, a beehive of activity. The boatloads of dead were deposited along the docks like the catch of the day, now at full capacity, the makeshift morgues further compounding the possibility of widespread contamination.

"Moroccan mayhem at its finest" proclaimed the admiral. "Alright, let's have a closer look."

The RIBs or Rubber Inflated Boats were launched in sequence from the George H.W. Bush. They approached the naval disaster, not a crime scene yet per se, but eerily reminiscent of the Titanic's fateful impact with a giant ice cube or sneak attack on Pearl Harbor that fateful Dec 7th morn back in 1941. Thousands of sailors thrashed about helplessly, target practice for the Japanese snipers or shark bait. Either way, the brave seamen were sitting ducks, as good as dead. Overhead a few USAF Raptors circled the scene of the inconceivable collision.

"My God! Sir, the vessels are total write offs! The spill… encompasses a wide swath. It's a Sea of Red." It's sinewy fingers reached out all along the break wall. What initially looked like fuel floating on the surface was in fact bright red blood from all the victims shredded by the virus, the rest ravaged by countless rows of hungry serrated teeth. The pilot fought back hard from puking into his visor. "There's very little sign of life" as he circled for another flyby.

"Roger that."

A massive morgue and treatment facility set up in a few empty warehouses along the port prepped for the worst. The rag tag team of local docs and medical students were inundated with remnants of hardy travelers. Many Muslim medical workers turned toward the Hassan II mosque for a prayer. The tallest in Africa, 7th highest in the world, towering 689' over the port like a silent, soothing sentinel. For most it was too late. Row upon row of wretches reduced to sinewy strips of flesh, entrails and bones like the latest Syndaver medical school simulators. But these were the real McCoys, McDonald's, Smiths and Jones. They couldn't keep up with the putrid overpopulation problem.

"Hang in there, help is on the way" said Dr Hussain, a former pathology professor at the local Has-san II Med School. He had oft read the reports in the New England Journal Of Medicine, etc about the dreaded disease round the bend. But now it was knocking on his doorstep, up close and personal.

He knew his students were eager, smart scientists, but he hadn't anticipated this. They were seriously outgunned and manned.

As the anesthetic and analgesics ran out, and in lieu of the US medical ships loaded with the good stuff, Dilaudid and other powerful morphine deri-vatives and vaccines. The last resort was to light up hookah pipes with a potent syrupy intoxicating concoction of tobacco to provide some relief. The CDC oft warned of toxic exposure to chemicals not filtered out by the water and the risk of infectious disease, even cancer, Professor Hussain poopooed the papers in a last ditch, desperate attempt to ease their pain and suffering. Many felt light headed, on gossamer wings he noted. Perhaps the powerful placebo of the Powerbull, a Red Bull flavor added in recent years had truly given them wings on their final ascent, or descent.

The top UAAMRIID specialist, the go to guy, Dr Bernie Gum, was about to board a plane for Papau and New Guinea to combat a recent outbreak of Kuru.

"Bernie something's come up. Your plane's waiting… on runway 49er."

"Aww come on commander, this's no laughing matter" insisted the doc defiantly. "No pun intended". The dreaded disease often labelled 'laughing sickness' due to shivers, tremors and outbursts of uncontrollable laughter. A form of "mad human disease' transmitted much like mad cow disease or bovine spongiform encephalitis. In this case the practice of cannibalism, or eating the dead tribal members during a funeral service. Per-haps the ultimate morbid form of flattery, not only mimic or ape the dead in mannerism, but not mind-ing their manners, consume every part of the dead. The prions in a tainted brain may remain dormant upwards of a decade or two, but ultimately mani-fest themselves after the macabre ritual. The survivors carry a resistant protein prion variant. “I’ve been waiting my whole life for a case such as this one.”

“There are a whole lot of lives at stake if we don’t nip this one in the bud” snapped the commander. “Millions!”

“Millions?”

“The fate of humanity squarely rests on our shoulders now Bernie. It’s in your hand’s son. We’re their last hope” pleaded the seasoned specialist. He was piling it on deep and thick he sensed. They had shared many a victory together. ”Failure is not an option!” The words resonated in his ears. Stirred him to his very soul. His eyes wide awake. They were oft called in as a last line of defense, USAMRIID’s last resort. “If that plane leaves the ground and you’re not on it, you’re gonna regret it, maybe not now, maybe not later, but soon and for the rest of your life." He paused… to see if the specialist was truly on his game, behind the eight ball.

"What God forsaken corner of the globe are you sending me to this time Chris?"

"Casablanca. No pun intended" he chuckled then regained his usual mean composure. "On a wing and a prayer."

"I'm on my way."

Eager to please and perhaps spend some time in one of his favorite film trivia locales. Rick's Ameri

-can Café.

"What can I get you?" asked the vivacious Virgin Airlines stewardess.

"Gin and ….surprise me." He peered at the pass-engers next to and across the aisle, each a drink in hand. "I feel like I'm three drinks behind" quipped Bernie. "If all the world leaders would just slow down and loosen up and have at least three shots we wouldn't need the United Nations."

The Virgin stew chuckled. "You'd better pace yourself." The long flight coupled with decreased oxygen pressure increases the effects of alcohol.

His failing marriage and the sultry Virgin vixen encouraged him even more to partake and forget his woes for just a while. He tried to keep his worst fears at bay. All the insidious little virus needed was a vector, a little nudge to send it leaping across the Pillars of Hercules straddling the Straits of Gibraltar to wreak a full scale attack upon the European mainland like the elusive Desert Fox, Erwin Rommel.

The foxy female hostess brought a tall frothy glass of Diamond gin fizz or French 75 dating back to WWI referring to the 75 mm field gun. In lieu of the carbonated water, a sparkling splash of wine. The unique additive, a raw egg yolk shaken and stirred vigorously. It added a smooth silky texture and flavor. In the mind of the medical maven it spelled salmonella. He summoned the stew with his forefinger.

"Uh miss."

"Yes? Is everything alright?"

"As a matter of fact… "I prefer my poison sans oeuf. Without the egg.." He whispered the word Salmonella in her ear.

"I'm sorry sir. How silly of me." She exchanged the drink for a tall golden delight. "The perfect drink for my favorite passenger" she said seduc-tively as she leaned into his cheek.

The deceptive concoction, the 'storm of the century' combined one oz of gin, light rum, dark rum, coconut rum, raspberry liqueur, triple sec, vodka, three oz of orange juice and a maraschino cherry on top. It took its toll almost immediately. He slipped into a comfortable sleepy comatose-like state and grabbed some shut eye. He knew she was trying to subtly seduce and have her way with him. Bernie suggested they meet over cocktails at Rick's Café upon safe arrival at their earliest opportune moment ere the elixir completely TKOed him.

"Ladies and gentlemen, this is your captain speaking. Please prepare for final descent into Casablanca." The flight crew was contacted re-garding the growing concern of the possibility of a full blown epidemic running rampant across the city. Mohammed V Int'l, a springboard to Europe, Africa, the Middle East and the Orient served some 7.5 million passengers/year. It was built in 1943 WWII by the Allied forces during 'Operation Torch' for the invasion of N. Africa. Odd how history has a funny way of repeating itself. The elusive entity had to be contained at all costs ere

it swept across the Saharan sands like a demented Desert Fox.

Bernie stepped from the plane rather light headed, on a date with destiny he hoped. The Virgin stew had stuffed her contact info into his leather flight jacket compartment. She meant business it seemed. They parted ways like two ships passing in the night. A row of small red cabs lined the arrival area. A vital vibrant artery surging through the heart of the city. The small red fiat whisked him toward the port district.

"The natives must be restless" he stated suspicious of the rising plumes of smoke above the harbor.

"Je ne sais pas" stated the cabbie shrugging his shoulders. He parked nearby. A swarm of masked men ushered the overwhelmed virologist inside the cordoned off warehouse. Their bloodied masks and haphazard hazmat suits prepped him for the shock of his life.

"Suit up!" He was hustled through the pale putrid compartmentalized sections much like a bio level 4 hazard facility. Each more menacing than the last.

"I had no idea. Just how bad is it?"

"Worse than the mask of the red death" snapped the senior resident facetiously eerily alluding to

Edgar Allan Poe's tall tale albeit not likely far from the truth. Their blood, sweat and tears now indis-cernibly oozing from each orifice.

"We waited after we dragged them from the sea. Rather than respond to aggressive therapies, it took a turn for the worse." A nurse collapsed inundated with the diorama of death all around.

"Gotcha." Bernie tossed her onto a gurney but in his experience it was already too late. Second chances were too few and far between. A second medic simply drew the red stained covers over her face. She looked like she'd cried a river of… blood emanating from every orifice ere she collapsed.

They hurried him to the dock and the source of the giant plume of smoke spotted for miles.. one of the morgues now designated a crematorium.

"We can't risk a burial, even at sea. " stated the senior resident on the verge of tears. The massive bilge pumps furiously sucked the toxic tainted film floating on the surface of the water into large storage tankers to avert further contamination. They served as floating crematoria incinerating

any possibility of transmitting Ebola.

The USNS Comfort, the length of three football fields, already filled over capacity; some 3 000 patients stuffed into the original bulkheads normally outfitted for 1000. "The problem with the obsolete hospital ship is each original oil bulkhead has no hatch, we have to lower them through hell exposing them again. We thought it would serve the sick better by isolating them."

"We were wrong. The hemorrhagic fever spread like a brush fire. "

"Hemorrhagic fever?" He stepped into his worst nightmare. "How do you know?"

The suited host entered a makeshift isolation tent and gently lifted the cover. Bernie froze in his tracks. "Why weren't we warned? Someone must have taken a hint! How did it get out of hand so fast?"

"That's what we can't figure out."

"It appeared as an all or none phenomenon."

"Where did it originate? Liberia?..."

"Liberia? International travel has been banned. Every African port is quarantined."

"The best of our sources suggest it originated on a ship."

"A cargo vessel?"

"Bigger. Cruise liner, the Mystique of the Seas, scattered about off shore as far as the eye can see."

“My God.” Bernie froze, trying to swallow the lump in his throat.

“Human… or… animal?”

“We believe it originated in a passenger, ironically air lifted from the vessel, about two weeks ago.”

“Two weeks?!”

“He’s hanging on by the skin of his teeth in intensive care in Cape Town. Said he was given a clean bill of health as he left Sierre Leone during the outbreak.”

“He must’ve come in contact with a few folks.”

“To say the least. That’s where it gets interesting…” as the senior surgical resident began to unravel the mysterious circumstances surrounding the escaped entity.

“We found this on the bridge.”

Bernie examined the water resistant smartphone loaded with selfies. A smiling captain next to a young blond haired woman and a few crewmen on the bridge.

"That's Will's fiancée."

"Will?" He thought last will and testament.

"Uh, the team leader for the MSF, Doctors Sans Borders." Bernie studied the photo carefully.

"Look at his eyes. The captain exhibits a transformation in color of the iris and cornea. Like albinism, a sign of immunological privilege or immunity."

"Privilege? This virus tore through the ship, it took no prisoners regardless of socioeconomic status, age, race or sex. Does this look like any of the upper class passengers had special treatment? We gave them all our best! Besides many victims from all walks of life exhibited the 'look'." He referred to the mish mash of iris-corneal pigments as he raised a few covers from the heads of a few victims. "They ALL exhibit a similar discolor-ation."

"He was the likely carrier. We discovered a case in which Ebola resides in immunologically privi-leged parts of the body - cartilage, semen or the eye ball."

"But how did it infect so many, so fast?"

"Close quarters, exposure to an infected host, tainted food, recycled water, sewage, waste..."

"We began to incinerate the deceased... try to contain it onboard and to the confines of the imme-diate area and morgues set up in a dozen warehouses on the dock."

"Tick tock" stated the seasoned specialist as he panned the perimeter. He watched the smoke rise high above the port. The plume could be seen for miles out to sea ere it dissipated over the Mediter-ranean. "Pray it isn't airborne.....yet."

The majority of survivors of the Pride of the Sea were isolated and transferred aboard the USNS Mercy, the respected sister ship of the Comfort. Some 4000+ saved souls.

"We're sending them back to Bethesda, Mass General, NYU, and a number of well equipped naval hospitals along the eastern seaboard."

"Not without an official clearance you're not."

"We caught it in time. There's every indication these folks will make a full recovery."

"We don't know what we're dealing with yet. A new strain perhaps? Why, even a clean bill of health doesn't amount to a hill of beans it seems these days" snapped Bernie disgustedly. Out of the corner of his eye he caught the crew of a small vessel, the RV Neil Armstrong sort through the sludge floating on the top of the water.

"It'll be one giant leap for mankind if we were to eradicate this entity entirely."

"One small step at a time" mused Dr Hatfield anxiously, from under his Tilly dirigible hat passed through the bowels of an Indian elephant several-times. "It's a veritable treasure trove. Like a paleontologist hired by a lucky lottery ticket holder to haul the winning numbers inked on a scrap of paper buried somewhere deep beneath the bloody layers of compressed pardon my French…shit." It stunk to high heaven. "The key to this carnage lies in there somewhere" mused the medical virologist.

He was usually right nine point nine nine nine nine times out of ten.

The large crane, like a nickel digger at the carnival hauled the mucky mess and deposited it onboard. It fell through a large grate in the aft deck to be sifted, sorted and analyzed for contaminants and trace elements, and clues. The bloody effluent swished and swirled about onboard.

"We'll leave no stone unturned" said a fellowship recipient proudly popped onto the deck in a hermetically sealed neoprene suit.

Bernie immediately noticed the redneck's inexperience. No protective gear other than medical grade gloves and a wet suit presumably an impermeable membrane. He feared the researcher could get exposed if he touched an infected surface.

"Hey, Jose can you see…watch out!"

"It's Charlie, Charlie Wilson. No relation to the Texas senator who single handedly brought an abrupt halt to the Afghanistan war."

"We're obviously in good hands" assured Bernie facetiously as the sharp metal edges of the pieces of the puzzle poked the curvy posterior of her tight neoprene membrane suit.

"Ouch."

"I hate to say I told you so, but….. Let me look at that."

"Hands off!" She snapped defiantly as she hurried under the glass encased outdoor shower to wash the enigmatic film from herself. Then slowly, provocatively unzipped the front of her suit to give a little sneak peek of the buried treasure. Bernie helped his charming coworker from her suit. She shook her head and unleashed a long golden mane of shoulder length strands.

She removed her gloves and shoved the suit to her waist. Her soaked underlying cotton body suit lapped up much of her perspiration. A small laceration in her arm and lower back alarmed the virologist. He applied salve and dressing quickly then gave her a jab. One of two experimental vaccines, an attenuated human Ebola virus reprogrammed to turn on itself to combat the common cold and live form of the virus. The other also an experimental anti cancer concoction, a double whammy.

"You've been exposed" he said earnestly. "No telling what's lurking in that slimy sludge."

"Thanks. I owe you one" she said as she wrapped her arms around him, then raised the visor for a quick peck on the cheek. Their lips locked, ere he could respond in his slightly inebriated state, a fatal faux pas feared Bernie.

"It's an acquired taste I know" she quipped licking her lime-tequila flavored lip balm to mask the stench of her habitual smoking.

"Are you crazy?" alarmed at the potential exchange of saliva.

"Crazy's my middle name. Have to be working with the mad hatter. After all, only he could convince me to dive into that cesspool teeming with tainted human corpses and toxic debris."

"She's one tough cookie" acknowledged the bearded captain. Like Ahab, in his relentless quest to capture the elusive great white… whale.

"Those that survived the impact were swallowed whole by an infestation of great white."

Bernie caught a glimpse of the dismembered, shredded appendages the scrubbers, pumps and cranes salvaged. He became sick to his stomach.

"I've never seen anything like it. Aye, it's the making of the perfect storm."

"Not a cloud in the sky, only a swirling particulate laden smoke cloud" noted Bernie as he leaned over the rail to hurl his airline snack.

"The admiral's about to announce to the world, 'Mission Accomplished'. Enemy contained. To the port of Casablanca. He's a damned fool. The blind leading the blind. He ought to know better. Have a look."

Dr Hatfield ushered Bernie toward one of the microscopes, the Ebola virus under the spot light on a carefully prepared slide.

"The unmistakable 'U', ' 9' or shepherd's crook" stared back at him ominously.

"By hook or by crook it always comes back with a vengeance, better prepared to fight our host defenses. It may've only been discovered within the last 50 years, but make no mistake this predator's been around lurking in the bushes since the beginning of time. Just like its toothy grinned partner in crime."

"Lighten up Larry" urged Charlie. "Or it's gonna eat you alive."

Bernie had the perfect segue to satisfy his cravings and kill two birds with one stone. "Speaking of food, I'm f…amished. Besides Rick's Café is right around the corner."

"Let me freshen up. I'll catch up with you." The quick change artist transformed from a surreal bloody stage prop to a tempting treat in tight casual jeans.

They approached the famed eatery, an uneasy tension in the air. Guests were carefully checked for ID at the door, a precautionary measure to prevent the possibility of infected riff raff from entering the premises.

The old courtyard style mansion, in the Old

Medina, typified the theme of the film. Its curved arches, balustrades and balconies, even the plants cast their eerie shadows against the white back drop.

The waiter seated them, and poured distilled water into their glasses. Bernie scoured the menu.

"American Crab, John Dory, with an eye spot on the side of its body fools its prey then snatches it with i's big mouth; and a house staple, Sole Meuniere."

"Fresh?" Bernie's words sliced through the tension like butter.

"Caught this morning right, right off the dock. Ere the 'event'" he said with a nervous whisper, and a wink downplaying the naval tragedy as best he could. All of the local shops and restauranteurs feared an economic fiasco if word got out about an Ebola outbreak. Tourism could grind to a halt.

A pianist's nimble fingers accompanied by a quartet began to tap a few chords. The innocuous beat of "What the hell I got?" inspite of the ominous insinuation, perhaps intentionally, it caught everyone off guard and uplifted everyone's spirits.

Hey baby on my mind

You're doing something to me every time

Too much and always stoned

I'm drinkin' baby drinkin' all alone…

The Virgin stewardess sauntered into the bar, out of uniform. She caught a glimpse of Bernie seated across from his captivating date she presumed. Her spiked high heels dug into the hardwood floor, spun a full 180 degrees about to storm from the premises.

"Claire, wait" shouted Bernie.

The stew eagerly awaited a plausible excuse.

"Excuse me. Prior plans."

"Claire. I'd like you to meet a few colleagues of mine. We're all in the same boat so to speak."

"Colleagues. Oh? She's not…"

"No, purely platonic and professional."

Don't know what the hell I got
Whatever it is it's an awful lot
Hey I'm gonna lose control
From my liver to my very soul
Yeah, yeah, yeah, yeah.

Claire joined the scientists, to even the playing field, now equally matched - two females, two males. The perfect foursome dinner date?

"I'll have a gin fizz and…" she said thirstily.

"Your sole" stated the waiter perfectly timed as he placed the aromatic golden brown dish in front of Bernie. "American Crab Louis." He placed the large salad plate in front of Charlie. Iceberg lettuce, the egg hard boiled, garnishes, Dijon mustard…all prepared by local food handlers. Bernie's worst fears resurfaced.

Suitcases in my hand
Packing baby, packin' all I can
Tunes rollin' in my head
Make me think of all the things you said

"In town for business or pleasure?" asked Claire politely.

"Work. Eight days a week" Dr Hatfield said off the top of his head.

"Well you know what they say, all work and no play makes Jack a dull boy" turning her attention to Bernie. She only had eyes for him.

"There's never a dull moment 'round here." snapped Charlie as she stabbed her crab meat.

The John Dory's eye on Bernie's plate stared back at him like a scorned spouse. The divorce was all but finalized. All that was needed was to ink and seal the deal. Soon he'd be a free man.

Don't know what the hell I got
Whatever it is it's an awful lot
Hey, I'm gonna lose control
From my liver to my very soul....

"Your gin fizz." A golden gin fizz to be precise. Bernie missed the fatal faux pas completely lost in Claire's eyes.

I don't want to be lonely
No, no, no, no, no
I don't want to be lonely
Lonely without love....

Claire sucked the gin, lemon juice, sugar, carbonated water and an egg yolk swiftly through the straw like the bilge pumps and scrubbers off shore. Likely suck a golf ball through a garden hose. The possibility of salmonella contamination remote.

Although, only a short hop, skip and a jump to the back door of the kitchen from the Ebola exposed docks stacked the odds against her astronomically.

Claire coaxed Bernie onto the dance floor. Such a clandestine encounter. 'Louis'… "I think this is the beginning of a beautiful friendship" said Bernie borrowing Bogey's immortal line from the film..

"I can't wait to get to know you" she said squeezing him tightly in her arms. Bernie reciprocated, for he too longed for the warm embrace missing in his life. It had been such a long time.

The song was interrupted with a short jubilant announcement.

"Sorry to interrupt folks, but I have some good news, word of a V-A day",. Bernie was not aware they had designated a day to honor the war veterans?" Victory in Africa' is imminent." Realistically they were weeks, maybe months or even years away from wading through all the waste and human remains harboring the feisty fugitive. Yet word spread through the dock district by by word of mouth from each flaming red cab as it raced through the streets like Paul Revere warning Bostonians the British were coming. It took the edge off of an impending economic chaos and collapse. The premature announcement could make matters worse if even the slightest oversight in procuring a clean bill of health prevailed.

"What did I tell yuh? Probably straight from the horse's…." he refrained from saying ass. The saying stumped a few Moroccans unfamiliar with the American slang. "I think we should be going." Charlie stuffed the last leaves of the iceberg lettuce into her mouth.

"Coming?"

"Go on. I won't be long…." declared Bernie obviously detained by his alluring dinner date.

"Early bird gets the worm" she replied. The double edged entendre sailed over his head, deeply pressed against Claire's cheek. He raised his arm and waved to his colleagues.

3: Cape of Good Hope

"Those that sow in tears
shall reap in joy."

- Psalm 126: 5-6 KJV

The port was restored to some of its former vibrancy, spirited trade and commerce after the smoke clouds dissipated. Moroccans were shuffling about, visiting their local hookah shops sharing tall tales of bravery and heroism after facing an insurmount-able foe. The only smoke trails now wafted from the frequented tobacco establishments. No one could foresee it might be merely the calm before the storm.

The massive slick, an assortment of human debris, naval fuels and other toxic fluids had allegedly been successfully contained. Incinerated in a flash with a potent upgrade of agent Orange coupled with a thermobaric bomb that sucked all the surrounding oxygen for a powerful blast. A raptor flyby visually confirmed the clearly demarcated perimeter. A mile in circumference, the orange red inflatable rubber ring ablaze circled the silent sea like a massive particle collider.

"We've rounded up and culled the herd" stated the fighter pilot flippantly.

Admiral Saunders peered through his binoculars and scoped out the fast and furiously leveled littoral combat operation zone. Only the massive dismembered, rummaged decks remained like the exposed ribs of a ravaged prehistoric dinosaur carcass. To him it was always a cut and dry win based on casualty count. A numbers game.

"Well I do declare you've done your due diligence commander. "

"When you have the entire Mediterranean fleet at your disposal, well need I say more."

"Give the orders. Move 'em out."

"Aye aye, captain." A military bugler accompanied the raising of a flag, the CVN 77's seal - an F 35 II Lightning, F 18 Hornet and TBM Avenger torpedo bomber surrounded by 1000 points of light representing a higher calling, serving the greater good and the thousands of souls saved by the ship not to mention the grace of God. Atop the flag, emblazoned in a bold red, white and blue 'Mission

Accomplished' They headed out of port, pending any unwanted uprising, for a short jaunt to their home base in Naples.

On board the Neil Armstrong, reams of data confirmed the collection of 99.9% of the bodies but not necessarily the virus.

"It leaves a lot to be desired for it does not account for 'marine consumption', primarily shark bait, plankton and smaller species in the food chain coral and simply lost at sea."

"Silent waters run deep…sir" offered Bernie. "No one knows what evil might be lurking not only just below the surface but free to roam from here to Rome, hell, to eternity."

Dr Hatfield concurred irritably.

"All's fair in love and war" stated Charlie.

"I've never seen such a complete and utter disregard for human safety. We're not at war, not in the conventional sense. Tell that to our elusive enemy. More crafty and cunning than the Viet Cong gorillas, Khmer Rouge and ISIS combined. There's no telling where the little beast will rear its ugly head. We'll uncover more 'killing fields'. Mark my words."

Charlie cast a stone cold glance Dr Hatfield's way. It sent a shiver down her spine.

"I'm with yuh" agreed Bernie. "That's why I have to bid you adieu. I'm off to Cape Town to find some answers, uh conduct a little reconnaissance of my own."

"A skirt in every port?" quipped Charlie facetiously.

"You were wearing jeans, Jordache. I do notice these things" stated Bernie with an eye for details.

"See yuh 'round."

"We'll hold the fort" alluding to the battle for Ft McHenry in Baltimore harbor, the last outpost defiantly defended against the British invasion. Their sheer resilience later inspired the national anthem, 'The Star Spangled Banner'.

"Shall we?"

Emma accompanied her private medical entour-age out onto the tarmac. Some of the sickest survi-vors were already cared for in the 'enhanced cargo handling' system aboard the converted C130 J Super Hercules.

"I can't wait to see him again."

"Parting is such sweet sorrow…"

"We've only been apart for the better part of six weeks, but it seems like a lifetime."

He studied her face underneath the clear plastic tent fabric. She wasn't in the clear yet.

"The eyes have it." Emma was not amused or open to a tempting tryst. Not now. Her fingers trembled slightly. Likely scarred for life having lived through the hellish nightmare. Her fair complexion, slightly sunburnt, typical for a fair maiden. She'd take the souvenir from the shocking events to the grave with her shared by no one but herself. An unfathomable marine 'Ripley's Believe it or Not' bed time story!

"I know we've been over this a thousand times, and I hate to drag you through the mud again, but is there anything you recall right up to the 'baptism' er dunking?

Emma entered a trance like traumatized state.

"My husband must've slipped something into my ….purse. I discovered it while rummaging through it just before the gala. I don't remember how else the syringe got there."

"But you do recall using it."

"I'm not an addict nor abuse drugs, if that's what you're implying."

"No. I'm suggesting that parting gift from your fiancé saved your life. It's the only logical explanation."

The airborne interrogation team tried to make sense of Emma's miraculous recovery. Clearly a carrier, like typhoid Mary who unwittingly infected 51 people, several families, killing three in NYC, Mamaroneck, Oyster Bay, etc. as a cook. She died after spending three decades in isolation. Worse than solitary confinement in prison presumed Bernie. He couldn't fathom a more horrible fate for her. Yet knowing how many passengers she had come in direct contact with, a certain death sentence awaited her. 'Ebola Emma' undoubtedly the cause of countless deaths aboard. The reasons clearly defined in the medical report. Unprotected sex with her fiancé, exchange of bodily fluids, semen, sweat, saliva. Both of them in direct contact with crew, food handlers, shop keepers, numerous tourists, in close proximity on the fateful evening on the dance floor. After the first flying fickle fist of fate was flung.... What were the odds? An infected host showing no signs or symptoms, harboring Ebola in his eye, struck, the blunt force trauma forcing the infected fluid out and about so freely? He entered the variables into the laptop data base. A medical first. The odds were astronomical against such a rare deadly transmission. Sheer ignorance, oblivious to the rapidity of attack of the new strain sealed the ship's fate. Dante's Inferno on the high seas. Bernie couldn't dwell on nor change what was.

He only hoped he could only prevent a frightening future recurrence.

"The word is mum" stated the pilot, slipping in under the radar as preestablished , not to raise awareness and the distinct possibility of a terrorist attack to steal the precious potential bioweapon.

The Super Hercules swung a wide circle around the perimeter of False Bay on final approach then touched down at Cape Town International. To avoid alarming the general populace by galavan-ting through any of the terminals, a heavy armed convoy greeted the plane. Humvees, armed person-nel carriers and ambulances quickly transferred the 'wounded' to New Somerset Hospital. The motor cade narrowly averted a calamity with a semi run-ning a red light. The truck driver dozed off then dove into a used car dealership. A few Mercedes burst into flames upon impact, licking at the license plates of the last humvee.

"Keep moving."

"By hook or crook. We're gonna get this gal to the hospital on time." As determined as a proud father delivering his expectant bride either to the altar or the OBGYN ward, he was true to his word.

Emma emerged from her tent, and bolted for the reception desk ere the staff reacted to the onslaught of seriously ill arrivals.

"Where is he?"

"Miss. Miss, please remain calm."

"Who?"

"Dr Chambers?"

"Dr Who?" She couldn't recall anyone on staff by that name.

"He's a patient here."

"Oh" said the puzzled night shift.

She scoured the screen, page after page of admittance records, names back a month.

"No one by that name. Sorry."

"Please, check your records. He came in by AMS about 6 weeks ago, from a cruise ship."

"Ah, here we are. Dr Will Chambers….." She paused as she read the words 'deceased'.

"Please have a seat."

Minutes turned to an hour…as she was forced to watch the veritable funeral procession. All the emergency exposures swept by Emma in and out of the waiting area like a tsunami. She was once again the only soul left.

A senior staff member, Dr Rogers, decided not to sugar coat the grim facts nor pass the buck on to a resident and asked Emma to follow him.

"Where are you taking me?"

He led Emma and her military entourage into a special quarantined area.

"I'm afraid Miss Chambers, your fiancé did not make it. Complications arose during surgery that were incompatible with life."

"Liars!"

"Miss. Please."

"He had the wind knocked out of his sails but Will was, uh is a fighter!" she said still in shock and disbelief.

"His 'infection' spread to his brain."

"Infection? Come clean with me Doc. We ALL know it's Ebola."

"Yes, his symptoms developed instantly. And inspite of his massive innocuous dose of vaccine, I'm afraid his body's immune system could not muster a defense."

Emma went out of her mind. Weeks of waiting. Now this.

"Why wasn't I informed?" The deadly tables had turned in some sort of sick ironical twist. A tit for tat. Cosmic kharma?

"We couldn't get through to the ship. All communication was lost. She was a ghost ship." There was something they were not telling her. Murder on the high seas? A massive cover up, a conspiracy?

Emma sunk into her chair….causing concern for the staff. In her infectious state…'Ebola Emma' had the potential to spread the virus everywhere. Everyone she came in contact with. The vaccine wore off weeks ago, yet miraculously gave her immune system the jump start she needed to give her a fighting, second chance.

They tranquilized her to ease the terrible recur-ring trauma. She'd lost everything.

"She's a flight risk." A person in her state is unpredictable. She could infect so many more. I'm afraid we're going to have to quarantine her indefinitely" were the last words to enter her ear-drums ere she fell into a deep sleep.

Even Bernie found the remedy a rather cruel form of punishment. A bitter pill to swallow. With the latest medical advances there must be a better alternative. He had to find a way… out….

A plan began to brew in his brilliant mind. He hadn't lost hope.

A week elapsed. Dr Gum was on rounds round the clock tending the sick, bombarded with all manner of military and experimental medical concoctions. The never ending inconclusive trials.

"I'm gonna get you out of here. I promise" as he reached inside the hermetically sealed tent and held her hand.

"Why? Why Will? Why us?" There was no plausible answer. A terrible twist of fate. When God rolls the dice it seemed there were always losers.

"I think the sea air'll do her a world of good" declared the CDC expert.

"I'll leave her in your trusted hands." I expect her back before midnight" said the stern nurse like a sorority den mother or concerned parent.

"Emma I have a surprise for you. We're going on a little field trip."

She assumed he meant some sort of code word for escape, freedom, flee.

The hospital van was filled like an assorted box of chocolates, recovering Ebola patients, alcoholics, sex offenders, HIV included, etc. all afflicted with some addiction or blood borne disease. Quite the combination. All given a clean bill of health and a second lease on life.

The van hugged the coast highway, toward its furthest destination. They passed Simon's Town on the edge of False Bay, a former naval base for two centuries, only a few idle cannons lined the forti-fications in the event of an attack that never came. The driver pulled over at the sign "Cape of Good Hope", the most SW point on the continent of Africa. The western boundary of False Bay. The sea spray and words invigorated the whole lot of patients if only as a placebo. A flash of genius crept into Emma's mind. She had to act quickly.

Bernie took her on a short stroll to observe the flora and fauna while the others rushed to the water's edge. The driver had dosed off.

"At least 250 species of birds" said Bernie ominously, so many possible vectors to carry the virus,.. "including penguins."

"All dressed up and nowhere to go."

Emma reflected on her unfortunate situation, from the moment the couple stepped onto the dance floor.

"Hold me."

"I have two left feet" joked Bernie.

"Shut up and dance with me!" she demanded.

The birds and bees stirred about. The sugar birds like tiny hummingbirds with long tails related to the Australian honey eaters flitted about the sweet nectar of the fynbos or 'fine bushes' and protea or species of 'sugar bushes'. Many plants were fertilized by the honeyeaters. The refreshing sea spray and stimulating fragrance filled their nostrils. Protea from the Greek god Proteus… the 'shape changer' able to do so at will. Bernie, lost in the moment, locked in her arms. Emma led from the start as she swirled him about ever closer to the van. Her modus operandi clear in her mind's eye and no other. She reached down to pick a few fragrant petals, cutting herself, instantly infecting the ubiquitous species.

"Ouch." Ebola waited for the hovering swarm to sip the sweet nectar, like the forbidden fruit in the garden of Eden. Then catch a lift, the poison passed onto the new host indefinitely replicating itself. Bernie felt a deadly airborne transmission of the virus was inevitable. In time every bird species would come in contact with an infected vector he feared . Spreading their seeds of destruction around the globe. The 'butterfly' or 'bird' effect as he relabeled it, a rose by any other name. … The future offspring, eating Ebola embedded in decay-ing carrion, consumed like the dead by the can-nibalistic tribes of New Guinea. The spread of the virus guaranteed. The fate of mankind hung in the balance.

"Walk this way." Her enticing swaying hips woke the groggy driver. He had no time to react. It was too late. Like a pouncing leopard that could not change it's spots. She smashed a dull edged souvenir from the water's edge on the side of his head. He sunk into his seat with a dull thud. Emma pulled the concealed revolver from the glove compartment.

"Are you with me?" asked Emma feverishly as she waved the gun at him. She shoved the uncon-scious driver aside brushing her infected hands against his exposed skin.

"Wait a minute…He's dead!" said Bernie checking the driver's pulse. Aid a known carrier and flee, face a firing squad or get left behind? He peered around the emptiness of land's end. The lesser of two evils, he chose to abet the fugitive.

"Everyone I touch dies" stated Emma in tears. Being a carrier, a blessing? Hah, it's a curse."

"Come on."

The other 'free willies' waved to the van. Their fate now hung in the balance, tempted to pet the pretty birds. The infected flock of 'sugar bush' eaters spread their wings and soared high above the Cape of Good Hope. The gruesome irony only grew some more as the 'cape crusader' pushed the pedal to the metal. To spread her seeds of false hope in a desperate last ditch attempt to regain some sort of sanity in her shattered topsy-turvy life.

"You didn't really think this through did you?"

"Shut up. I'm not going back. Ever. Ebola Emma? My a…!" Her perceptiveness innate or likely acquired during her long prior relationship with the Medecines Sans Frontier. She knew what she wanted and obviously how to get it. Bernie was the perfect pawn, the next move his? Or hers in the growing global chessboard or game of battleship.

"All the world's a stage" he said nervously. The words resonated with Emma. She'd heard it all before from all the other suitors. But Will and Bernie were different. There was no BS, no sugar coated lies. They simply stated the truth. It was something she sought so desperately. Perhaps it was the only reason she hadn't pulled the trigger yet and fled in isolation. She needed him as much as he needed her. She for the elusive cure, the answer he sought. He, the golden ticket, to escape from the tightening noose around her neck, this never ending roller coaster ride. She felt her life spinning totally out of her control at this juncture.

All the excitement got the better of her as she passed out. Her limp form slumped over the steer-ing wheel. The van veered erratically across the road as her lead foot fueled the fiasco. Bernie grabbed the wheel and brought the vehicle to an abrupt stop. He could not feed Emma any more 'false' hope, as they sat by the dock of the bay of the same name. Harbor a fugitive, a carrier of the most insidious invader on earth, and risk global spread of the contagion, even his own death, was not his first choice. He had to call a couple coll-eagues, cash in on a few favors. Besides they owed him big time. The names of a handful of research-ers on Marion Is. midway between S. Africa and

Antarctica came to mind. He feared isolating her at the Ross Island research station that could trigger an Ebola epidemic of epic proportions amongst some 2 million Emperor penguins. The thought of a million females laying an egg susceptible to Ebola infection spreading to the seal and whale population or simply drift off, 'Ebola on ice' could have a far worse effect ultimately reaching landfall on every continent.   He perished the thought.

The Seychelles came to mind. Exiled on a sparse-ly populated rock, a remote tropical isle might not be so bad , just what the doctor would order for the both of them. Essentially disappear off the grid. Some serious R and R. Time to let some old wounds heal. Daring to boldly go to the British Indian Ocean Territory seemed a bit of a stretch. Diego Garcia, the largest southernmost island, now the site of a US Naval base and Strategic Air Com-mand and Military Sea Command responsible for replenishing naval forces' supplies did not sit well with him. She'd likely be dissected, sliced, diced and ultimately sacrificed for her bioweaponizable potential. He couldn't let the army get a hold of the cure first, not without unravelling it, studying it, replicating it. He linked via several southern hemi-sphere sitcom networks and cashed in his trump card. His career was on the line. Was he doing it solely for altruistic purposes? Or was there more to it? Was it love?

"Sam? Long time no see."

"See no evil, hear no evil, speak …of the devil."

"Say can I ask a favor of you?"

"For you anything, just name it."

"I happened to be in the neighborhood."

"You're in Madagascar? Haven't you heard, I relocated. A great opportunity came up to pursue that cancer research… Got a big US government over seas grant and all."

"No shit?"

"Came out smelling like a rose, no pun intended, after that containment breach back at the CDC."

"Caused quite the scare."

"I'm afraid we're in the same leaky boat, my friend."

"I can send you a couple airline tickets stat."

"It's not that simple."

"What have you got yourself into this time?"

"Deep shit. I'm at the Cape."

"Cape Cod?"

"Cape of Good Hope. Change in flight plans, a slight detour."

"Say no more, I 'll have a buddy, a fly fisherman with some time to kill at the Cape pick you up in his DeHavilland."

"I'll leave a smoke signal."

Bernie hurriedly staged their escape, ie 'death'. "Rings, give me your jacket, backpack." His tilly hat, extra pair of jeans etc. placed in the passenger seat.

He removed the gas cap, stuffed a hose in the tube and sucked. The gasoline burned his lips. He filled a jerry can with gas and doused the van ere he slammed it into drive and hurled the lit pack of matches across the front seat. Bernie shoved it off in a low budget christening. The vehicle burst into flames as it went over the rocky shoulder and down the embankment to the water's edge in a blaze of glory.

There were a few holes in his alibi, but felt, they'd call off the search in time. Driver's suicide, burned beyond recognition. The others escaped on foot without food, water, exposure to the elements disoriented, in a state of confusion. They didn't have a clue. The two of them, presumed dead, drowned or simply vanished? The possibility of a terrorist kidnapping or abduction also crossed his mind.

The couple savored the roaring campfire for a short time ere they heard the loud twin prop, twin pontoon relic sputter and splash down.

"G 'day mates. I'm Gus. Ain't she a beaut?" said the crusty seaplane pilot as he flipped the door and hopped off the restored 'King Beaver' or 'one ton truck'; the US Army, the largest operator of the aircraft.

"We've got a long flight ahead of us. Come on."

Bernie reached 'round Emma and hoisted her as if carrying her over the threshold. In this case, a wobbly, rusty, aluminum bucket of bolts.

"Pretty petunia, your wife she is."

"Uh, she's not my wife."

"Could've fooled me. Didn't take your eyes off her once."

"She's special. One of a kind."

Emma smiled, stirred by his soft spoken words or the vivid images in her weary subconscious. The cape crusader had a glimmer of hope and real freedom for the first time.

The treacherous 3900 mile trek at the best of times. They hugged the coastline on the first leg, then a hop, skip and a short jump for the flying jalopy from Lesotho to Swaziland and across the channel to Madagascar and virtual freedom. The rough flight unlike the hospitable Virgin experi-ence was marked by several scheduled stops to refuel always under the radar and watchful eyes of the authorities. They'd undoubtedly catch wind of their daring escape or untimely disappearance soon enough. Either way, the army would certainly track them down like wild animals. Grab and gut Emma then unravel and clone the elusive vaccine's for-mula for their arsenal of bioweapons; ever ready in the event of a clash with communism or any other rogue faction or terrorist regime.

Several tense moments seemed like an eternity as the plane sputtered over the unique spiked project-ions on the island. The towering sharp serrated edges of the weathered rock formation or Tsingy could grate the plane to pulp. Spark plugs would fly.

"Let's take a walk on the wild side" quipped the venturesome vet fumbling with the fuel mixture. As if he could ever top his death defying aerial act.

"Definitely not as inviting as the Dreamwork's classic."

He set his bearings NNE and bore down on the capital. His flight plan seriously in question as he soared over the rooftops of the thriving metropolis.

"I left my heart in Antananarivo" he sung off key. Above the bright city lights Emma and Bernie feared they were about to nose dive like a couple of stray cats onto a hot tin roof. "Over there." A large black heart shaped spot appeared. "An artificial lake in the middle of the city built by none other than James Cameron."

"Spare us the Hollywood Aviator's trivia" stated Bernie expecting a bitter end after a fiery crash.

"That's the other James Cameron. No relation to the …film producer." He eased off the throttle, narrowly missing the WWI Memorial in the center of the lake and a wingtip then set her down. He coasted to a stop at the opposite shore startling a flock of great egrets. Four species are found in all four corners of the globe.

"Egrets!" .

"None" said Bernie above the sputtering prop. "If you live life right once is enough." He could not conceivably relive or retrace the steps in the convoluted trail he had survived thus far. Oft a trailblazer, but always a leader never a follower.

"I think he meant egrets, not regrets" laughed Emma nudging him.

"How we ended up at the Grand Hotel I'll never know." Built by the Eiffel engineers, the quaint gardens and comfy rooms were most welcome.

"Relax, it comes with the territory, part of the perks of being a rock star scientist" boasted Barry, burning through his startup capital like campfire kindling. He'd picked them up in the hotel limo off the Rue Titsy, slightly tipsy from the trying voyage. The researcher hustled them through the park, aptly named 'Independence Place' to the main entrance of the Grand Hotel Du Louvre.

"I'm sure you could use a hot shower or a bubble bath" he said to the trio. His eyes locked mischievously with Emma's. Her warm radiating smile priceless like the Mona Lisa on display in the other Louvre. Admired by some 9.7 million annually, # one in the world. Emma by contrast was one in a million, in a league all her own, such a rare sight, worth her weight in gold in fact as the researchers would soon discover.

"When in Ant.. anana….ana… treated like royalty!" Diametrically opposed to the nightmare she'd lived through.

"It hasn't always been a cake walk or a walk in the park if that's what you mean."

"A toast to friendship."

"To friends….No ship. Ship is taboo."

"No shop talk tonight, agreed?"

They spent hours exchanging enchanting tales of their escapades, narrow escapes and close encounters.

"I'm bushed."

Emma dropped like a sack of sh….andeliers. The touch of the smooth silky sheets tingled at first like an immune response after a bee sting or all-ergic reaction to a foreign fabric. She dozed off deader than a door knob. It had been the first sound sleep in weeks. Bernie feared his sleeping beauty wouldn't wake for a thousand years yet refrained from entering her room and eased his fingers from the door knob.

4: Bright Eyes

"You put de lime in de coconut
And drink 'em bot' up."

- Coconut lyrics, Harry Nilsson

The alarm blasted. Bernie fumbled with the snooze button to no avail. The buzzing noise startled Emma who awoke from a dream, startled fearing for her life. An ambush? To send her life into another tailspin? Her head shot up into a pros-trate position. Bernie brought her a fresh pot of roasted coffee. Emma let the savory aroma of an African, Arabica blend permeate her nostrils. She

sweetened the simmering black gold with some brown sugar and took a few sips. It was just the jump start she needed to begin the day like any other.

Barry arrived in an older Jeep Wrangler Africa.

"Hey bright eyes" said the chipper colleague.

"I like your hot wheels."

"Steel wheels, 2.8 liter diesel. She'll take a bite out of anything Madagascar's off the beaten path can throw at us."

"No doubt."

They swerved through early morning traffic across town to the Medical School at Ambohit-saina. The Wrangler pulled up the long curved driveway. The site was concealed under a rich treasure trove of lush semi tropical vegetation.

"It looks like a miniature buried Mayan temple"

"Gimme shelter" commented Emma. bright-eyed and bushy tailed.

"As you wish."

They whisked her under cover of the rich green foliage and marched through the main building, one of only three visible, to an adjoining set of labs.

"Here we are. Home sweet home. For the last couple of years anyway."

A vast network of coiled, glassware, Erlenmeyer flasks , bunsen burners looked like a sophisticated mouse trap. "The best that money can buy. Thanks to the good ole USA grant."

"I'm impressed" stated Bernie at the fully equip-ped set up on par with any east coast Ivy League Organic Chemistry dept.

"It gives me pure VCR by the boatload."

Emma looked around. She saw neither a VCR or TV for that matter in the mad scientist's lair. Only microscopes, chromatography apparatus, laptops and computer screens filled with con-voluted ring structures.

"VCR?"

"Uh, that's Vincristine. A vinca alkaloid synthe-sized from the Catharanthus Roseus plant. It grows all over the place round here."

The words sounded vaguely familiar to Emma.

"Cath…Rose?…Refresh my memory."

"Periwinkle, bright eyes, 'old maid'."

"I'm not dead yet" she snapped facetiously.

She wandered around the intricate glass network watching a few drops of condensate wind through the glass coils and tubes until a few precious drops fell into a flask. Barry delicately picked it up and observed the clear color then swirled it around like a fine wine.

"Good to the last drop. Like a coveted fragrance. Worth every pretty penny."

"I'm sure" inquired Emma imagining splashing a jeroboam sized bottle of Chanel #5 or even rarer Amouage all over her body.

"$6000 an ounce."

"Why, you could start a lucrative grow op of sorts."

"I did. Made a half mil my first year. Completely legit. No bureaucratic red tape, other than throngs of infected tribesmen clamoring for the stuff during clinical trials. There's never enough to go around. And other than the usual vomiting or diarrhea, hair loss, etc. there are No unwanted side effects …like 'death' from cocaine or heroine abuse . Saves lives too, tens of thousands every year to boot, dying from cancer, childhood leukemia, Hodgkin's lymphoma, even lowers blood pressure. Rather than the senseless slayings, the cocaine cartel killing fields. No running from the law…"

"Until we arrived" joked Bernie.

"The best of both worlds really. Mind you, it takes 15 tons of petals to synthesize the miracle essence to produce 1 oz ."

"30,000 pounds."

"That is, the 10% of the useable part of the plant, the petal, the rest is discarded. Follow me." He led them into a steamy spacious greenhouse under cover of the dense vines and underbrush weaving over the glass enclosure.

"It keeps the direct sunlight out. Lets the flowers bloom. A new hybrid. I've been tweaking the amount of VCR I can squeeze from every petal."

"Like a mad medicinal marijuana scientist, up the cannabidiol percentage to relieve the epileptic seizures and cancer pain, reduce the THC and the addictive effects are lowered."

"Sort of. It's a juggling act, a fine tight rope high wire act. …You do seem to know your drugs."

"Product of my environment, uh former fiancé, doc, virologist."

"Ah…, so you see there is a method to my madness."

"Where do you harvest so many flowers?"

"The hills are alive with the sound of countless Malagasy periwinkle planters and pickers. 7 of the 8 strains known are indigenous to the island. The meter tall plants grow best in wooded areas, by roadsides on the slopes from 2500 to 6500 ft. We've edged out China with a little over 2 million pounds of petals per year."

"Amazing."

"The government doesn't mind?"

"Mind? They're onboard big time. One of the island's largest exports along with coconuts, tortoise shells and guano."

"No shit?" mused Bernie.

"The government fully endorses it?"

"It's the army I'm worried about. Like any drug, legal or illicit. If there's a profit to be made…"

"Build it and they will come" feared Bernie

"They've come knocking before."

"Can't you just uproot and relocate?"

"When the lease or the grant expires, whichever comes first."

"The old proverbial chicken and egg……huh?"

Barry's demeanor quickly changed.

The University of Antananarivo's chancellor was making his rounds, nosy as usual to see what Barry was up to.

"What's cookin' doc?" he quipped.

"I've asked a few colleagues to assist me in the experiment."

"The more the merrier. I'm predicting a bountiful harvest this year, no doubt."

Always eager to push the envelope or open it like stockings hung by the chimney with care, and stuff the green stuff, the endless royalties, that filled the campus coffers.

"You know I've been hearing nothing but good things from the joint venture we launched last year. Keep up the good work." Barry waited 'til the administrative brass' heckling and hen pecking was done for the day.

"Emma, you don't mind rolling up your sleeves?

"It looks like this place could use some elbow grease" she said facetiously, nervously awaiting the 'prick'

"You are the reason why we're here" he said preparing to aspirate the elusive additive that added years to her life.. We're risking our careers."

"Not at all."

"Shall we?"

Barry double gloved and suited up. He carefully forced the syringe into her forearm and drew the precious life saving liquid.

"I hope to identify all the trace compounds and elements of the vaccine circulating in your system that essentially saved your life."

"It's a mystery to me. I thank God I'm alive."

"Perhaps combine the vaccines in trial runs for a double whammy."

"Kill two birds with one stone?" joked Bernie.

"Yes, take on cancer with VCR, and as we discovered recently VCR packs the most potent punch against EVD or Ebola Virus Disease. The fast and furiously replicating cells of cancer and Ebola are extremely susceptible to VCR because it attacks the tiny microtubule formation which builds cells. It creates a real 'roadblock' so to speak."

"Like the futile attempts by the Narcs or DEA trying to capture and detain the head honcho of the cartels?"

"Yeah, sure."

"Where did you say you found her?"

"Shipwrecked off Casablanca."

"No!"

"She's the one" said Barry. His greatest fear, theft, a few syringes or vials slipped from the lab, down the food chain, unregulated use of the drug by black market thugs or junkies. It was likely traded for gold by them to medical staff and health organizations running out of options.

"You're beginning to creep me out, sound like the Matrix. Don't you dare ask me to take a blue or the little red pill, ha, ha?" she asked.

"No worries. VCR or Oncovin, the generic name, is only in injectable form."

"I suspect a variant of it was what your fiancé might've given you" as he held Emma's hand. Emma was startled. Was she the missing link? Merely a coincidence that she had come all this way? Cosmic kharma?

"It's highly toxic and site specific. 100% lethal if administered directly into the spinal fluid. That's why I'm worried, junkies 'll kill themselves. OD mistaking it for street drugs. It takes only a few micrograms to increase the survival rates of count-less cancer patients dramatically from 10 to 90%. I'm hoping it will have the same consequences against our elusive little friend,"

"Here's hopin'" said the good sport as she crossed her fingers following the procedure. Barry had filled several test tubes to begin the tedious blood analysis process to confirm the presence of the potent cure.

Barry shoved the test tubes into his lab coat as another loud series of knocks on the door echoed through the lab muted by the dense foliage of the greenhouse.

A team of armed militia stormed the lab.

"There she is. Get her."

"The cat's out of the bag."

"Come on. In through the out door."

He raised an inconspicuously covered trap door, a secret back exit under a section the garden undetec-ted by the roving surveillance cameras. They rushed down a 'fire escape' like ladder into an adjoining tunnel.

"Come on. This way" urged Barry as the blind led the blind out into the daylight.

Several rail tram cars were parked on the inclined slope. The descent into the endless sea of pink periwinkle petals all around stirred Emma.

"Periwinkle fields forever."

"Which one?"

"This one." The tram whisked them to a crossing where a Malagasy worker had pulled his African Wrangler around.

"Thanks Baba Looey" ironically named after Quick draw McGraw's faithful Mexican sidekick cartoon character.

"It's alright."

Barry slammed the diesel into drive. The sturdy steel wheels bore the brunt of the off road beating. The high torque engine spun the 35 inch mud terrain tires around the jungle like campus.

"Gus? Gus?" are you there?"

The groggy pilot awoke from his siesta, a high noon nap.

"Start your engines." He sprang into action and fired up the 'King Beaver' then taxied from the WWI Memorial parking spot in the center of Lake Anosy.

Barry bolted through the side streets in an effort to lose the military convoy in hot pursuit.

He raced toward the water's edge in 'Independence Park' and hustled his imminent exiled entourage onto the pontoons.

"This place looks vaguely familiar. Déjà vu?"

"Last night. Looks are deceiving during the day" acknowledging all the back stabbing campus and police security, not to mention the obnoxious military thugs always wanting a handout or payoff.

"Howdy partner." Gus' toothy grin spread across his unshaven, unkempt attempt at a full bearded Grizzly Adams look.

"Are we glad to see you."

The Beaver leapt from its watery enclosure and veered low due north over the outskirts of the capital to avoid any AirMad or military air traffic.

Several stray shots whizzed by the windshield. The military jeep unleashed several more rounds erratically if only to scare and bring them down in one piece.

"You fools! I need the girl, alive!"

Gus weebled and wobbled but wouldn't let the plane veer from its course heading due north.

"They're firing at us!" screamed Emma.

"Consider this my walking papers" sighed Barry.

The Indian Ocean lay ahead as far as the eye could see.

"Here we go again."

"Like I said I think it's time to leave the bright lights of the big city behind and branch out. Take our business, accounts and all, off shore. Besides you know how I hate hostile takeovers."

"Tell me about it" concurred the USAMRIID vet. Every step he took, monitored, scrutinized, under the watchful eye of a higher in command. He never could spread his wings and truly fly. He was not a free bird, not yet.

A few military aircraft, former fourth and fifth generation US hand me downs were in hot pursuit.

"Step on it Gus!"

"I'm slappin' the beaver as hard as I can" he yelled as the seaplane entered international waters. As far as the eye could see, not a palm tree or sliver of cover.

"Over there" noted Bernie.

"You're seeing things. We're nowhere near home plate" shouted Barry as the unmistakable illusion

formed on the distant horizon.

"Locusts?"

"No… bigger." The AirMad aerial armada veered away violently in the heat of the moment. A squadron of MQ9 Reapers swooped by narrowly averting a midair collision with the Beaver.

"What the sam hill?" said Gus in disbelief as he rubbed his bloodshot eyes.

"Making their rounds" reassured Barry sweating bullets.

"Just how do you plan to continue your cancer research out here, research vessel disguised as a trawler or tuna boat?"

"Hmmm." Barry mulled. They'd escaped by the hair of their shinny chin chins. This continuous charade, dodging the bullet either by administrative Russian roulette or militia firing squad came to

a boil.

Gus entered the Seychelles chain of some 115 Islands over 1000 miles from the northern edge of Madagascar.

"I'm starved" said Emma. Skipping breakfast did not sit well with her. The most important meal of the day… oft left to chance these days.

"Mahe?"

"Mahi, mahi? I love the sound of that. I don't mind a hearty brunch."

"The main island. There's a couple of great seafood restaurants in Victoria.

"Can't wait."

The water taxi veered over the pristine pictur-esque tropical island. Victoria the capital, lay to the north east comprised of a about a quarter of the 90,000 islanders.

He taxied over the small port and sought Barry's 'houseboat'. All transfers were by stevedore or dock worker manual labor. Gus pulled the plane next to the "Fisherman" in honor of Zane Grey's yacht.

"Ah home sweet home."

"Paradise ladies and gentlemen."

" Exports include vanilla, coconuts, fish, soap and guano."

"No shit?" A peculiar musty odor came across the starboard bow.

"We're gonna need a bigger boat. … to haul the petals and vaccines across the pond."

"Miles ahead of you." He pointed to the large tanker presumably the source of the awful stench.

A large tugboat sat in a neighboring berth.

"Used to transfer the bags of guano from the mines."

"Bat shit?"

He nodded.

"Bird droppings. More than a million tons

give or take in the last century alone. Some of the best organic fertilizer on the planet." Barry con-tinued. His audience spellbound plugging their noses. "During the last ice age, the entire bird population from the northern hemisphere sought refuge in the subtropics. Five of the islands were hardest 'hit'. Providence. Piled 50 feet deep, scraped some 160,000 tons off the surface of Assumption. Astowe 70,000 tons, St Pierre and Denis Islands.

"That's a load of crap! I suppose you're gonna tell me that's how the term PhD came about."

"No, he's right" concurred Bernie.

"The bat scrapings were up to a meter thick, oft blasted from the caves. Then sorted, mixed and left to dry. The rail cars brought them to shore. Then manually bagged up to 120 boatloads per day. The government received a royalty or leased the land to businessmen.

"Well it's gonna take a lotta guano boats to haul the rosea petals from here to commercially viable synthesizing center."

"2 million plus pounds. 10 percent of the plant is usable petals from which to extract the VCR."

"Let's not jump the gun. We have a hard row to hoe. Analyze the results. Begin trials."

"We may not have time to take this to clinical trials. When they drag us into a court of law let alone in front of a firing squad" feared Bernie.

"My guys at UGib are waiting for the first samples."

"UGib? You're not jib jabbing me are you?"

"University of Gibraltar. The 'joint venture' the chancellor was referring to. Opened their doors back in '15. A cooperative agreement with USey uh University of Seychelles established in '09 sealed the deal. The US funded the first of its kind global venture to combat cancer. .

"You don't say?"

"I do say. USey. You see?"

Barry was tongue tied, thirsty after their narrow escape. "Can I get you anything….?"

"A valium" said Emma edgy, nearing her time of the month they sensed.

"To drink?"

He pushed a metal cylinder into a coconut then pounded it a few times with a wooden mallet like a judge silencing a courtroom. Then generously poured a splash of gin and lime into all of the open ended containers except Emma's while singing the song, 'coconut'.

"You put de lime in de coconut and you drink 'em 'bot up…."

In turn, he handed a coconut to each colleague.

"Bottom's up."

"Mmmm" said Emma as she lapped up the luxurious virgin liquid.

"It's a breeze."

"If"

> "French fries kill more people than guns and sharks yet no-body's afraid of French fries."
>
> - Robert Kiyosaki, Hawaiian born US entrepreneur, author 'Rich Dad, Poor Dad'

The new surround sound speakers cranked out a steady beat that drove the crowd into a frenzy.

"14,000 watts of pure pumping power, 300,000 watts of decadent delight…uh lighting."

"What?" quipped the DJ testing the new sound system at Es Paradis. The reno a vital part of the strategic revitalization of the club district nestled near the vibrant small fishing port of San Antonio on the island of Ibiza. The wide eyed skimpily clad waitresses noshed on a few French fries ere their busy shift began that inaugural evening. The blazing bewildering light show coupled with a few unique new fun filled party treats was a sure fire way to draw the dapper decadent crowd from as far as Mallorca, Minorca Barcelona and the French Riviera. The high rollers, happy go lucky honeymooners, and night owls alike.

"It's going to knock their socks off! No pun intended" said the suave Spanish entrepreneur proud of his tempting discotheque. The posters were splashed on all the adjoining streets.

"Paint party?" The skimpily clad vixens frolicked about covered in a decadent rainbow of colors.

"Come on. It's the talk of the town" urged a venturesome vixen to her shy boyfriend dragging him to the center of the traffic circle. "Don't be a chicken Pedro!" she quipped as he crossed the road and sought shelter under the giant 'egg'. The swel-tering noon day sun coupled with her unbeatable return serves had pooped him out on the court.

He admired the mini replica of the Santa Maria inside the cavernous hollow center of the massive egg, 'Christopher Columbus' Egg. Allegedly named after the venturesome explorer, first to set sail and discover the new land. His trip fortunately funded by a harmless bet. The nobility had asked the simple question, 'How is it possible to stand an egg upright without falling over?' The winner will received the funding he seeks. Countless attempts to balance the wobbly oblate spheroid shell on the king's table were made. They were stumped, at a loss, all gave up except one conniving Chris-topher Columbus, neither a man of means or family fortune. He held the egg for a moment, then gently tapped the end with a silver spoon. Colum-bus then placed the egg on the table where it remained in an upright position. The funding was his.

"If you can answer this riddle I'll accompany you to the club" he said mischievously.

She mulled over it for minutes ere she threw her arms in the air and gave up.

"Tell you what lover boy, if you accompany me to the club and pop the question in front of my friends I'll make this the most unforgettable evening of your life."

"Done."

The couple disappeared in a sea of similarly dressed in decadent transparent attire revealing speedos and other flimsy forms of g string or dental floss bikini under garments.

"I'm sorry. Dress code clearly states respect-able attire. Swimwear to be worn underneath."

"Aww come on."

"No ifs, ands or buts" said the stocky bouncer as he eyed the luscious caboose and under carriage of Pedro's girlfriend.

"But I'm only in town for a night on a layover" said the steaming stew.

"Change, then come back."

The stewardess huffed and wandered into a club with a far less demanding club before puffing out of breath.

The alluring lights and loud music fired up the feisty audience, foreigners and locals alike.

The gyrating bodies in sync to a steady beat. As if the eye candy was not enough, Es Paradis quickly kicked it up a notch. The outer garments were soon shed. A handful of seductive staff, waitresses who agreed to work overtime or even on their off days faced off. Armed with harrn-less squirt guns and pistols, they awaited the word with baited breath.

"Fire!" The colorful stream of neon glow shot from each weapon like a flame thrower. Their bodies soon aglow in a dazzling display of brightly glowing day glow paint.

"I said Paint! Not 'fire' you fool!"

Unfortunately amidst the confusion, some had erroneously mistaken the word 'fire' for a more immediate threat. Many clubbers headed for the exits. In the ensuing stampede many bodies were tramped. Those fortunate to flee in the first wave beelined straight for the beach. The water was too tempting. No one needed to peel off their clothes. Covered in the colorful, camouflage, that could actually be seen for several blocks or the neighboring rooftops created an instant spectacle. A bizarre colorful water ballet ensued. The thrashing and splashing soon alerted a school of roaming great white who had ventured into the port. The erratic motion coupled with a cascade of colors must've appeared like a lucid LSD trip for the ecstatic sharks. The countless feeding mach- ines who had feasted and gorged in a furious frenzy on the victims of the Mystique sought to continue the killing spree. An encore now inevitable.

The laughter turned to blood curdling screams that echoed through the fishing port. The razor sharp serrated edges bore down on the bright neon painted bodies. It was a sight for sore eyes, even the partially blind. The painted ladies discarded their bottles of wine. Their bodies unmistak-able homing beacons in the night. A horrific nightmare ensued.

A bright red tint instantly over rode the other primary colors. To seemingly add insult to injury in the macabre feeding frenzy, a swarm of vultures Pharoah's chicken, ISIS chosen converged to challenge the marine monsters for the best selection in the San Antonio smorgasbord. There was no escape from the hellish nightmare, either above or below the surface.

Several crazed travelers sought to put an end to

the endless screaming by putting the victims out of their misery and clubbed them like helpless seals.

Pedro rushed from Es Paradis or 'Paradise', out into the streets. The mad crowd, in utter disarray and states of dismemberment panicked and dashed down the streets helter skelter screaming.

"Sofia?" yelled Pedro.

"So many!" shouted a crazed partier, partly deafened by the mind boggling roar, mistook as 'so few.'

As a last resort he bolted toward the traffic circle at the entrance to San Antonio in a desperate attempt to find Sofia. He observed the panic stricken clubbers, now displaying an additional bright red camouflage. The mere stench of the crowd drew the Canary Island vultures out in droves. The birds swooped down like spitfires pecking at the bloody flesh on each flyby.

"Back to the egg" he said or thought out loud. It made no difference in the mindless menacing air raid. He followed the curve of the giant egg shell.

"Sofia?"

He grabbed on to the female form clutching the masts and intricate rigging of the miniature Santa Maria in a complete state of shock.

"Santa Maria!" she repeated over and over.

"Sofia!" he shook her. She snapped from her near catatonic state. She'd lost a lot of blood. He had to act fast to get her to the nearest emergency dept. Did the island even have a hospital he wondered, likely overrun by now.

"Lights out?" snapped a few retirees as they clapped to turn out the lights in their flat. They perused the darkened port unaware of the blood bath. The screams had subsided. The colorful glowing display coincidently reduced to a dull lifeless sea of red as they clapped. The second and third wave fiercely fought off the remaining black tipped vultures ere they flew away in search of more islands to pluck.

"Flock off!" yelled the club owner angrily as he peered about, his livelihood and island lay in ruin.

The growing menace of great white egressed like the tide then headed to pillage and plunder the beaches of the Balearic Islands like the Barbary pirates of old. A state of emergency was declared as the ERs were overrun. Ebola intent on destroying everything in it's path in the sneak attack.

"Watch your step" said the tour guide as the last of the group seated themselves in the tiny vessels scattered about the bizarre landscape. The gaudy garish grimaces and shadows cast off the massive stalactites and stalagmites ablaze in a glow of black light lit colors inside the cavernous space was mind blowing.

The music, a complete Bach and Beethoven movement and overture. The concert resoundingly echoed from deep inside the underground acoustic chamber. Truly, a one of a kind performance. Cuervo de Drach, or Dragon's Cave off the coast of Mallorca. A loud standing ovation followed the movement. A sudden erratic sound like a flutter of a swarm of bats or birds over-whelmed the audience. They fought frantically to defuse the enraged swarm. Their arms, ideal targets for the tiny claws and fangs swinging over their heads.

The enraged fruit bats continued to pierce the skin, and lap up the luxurious liquid. Their tainted blood exposed to Ebola but a few days ago during a feeding frenzy in one of the numerous seaside caves. Several bodies that had washed ashore, later identified by the local authorities, carried off by the currents from the fateful cruise off Morocco. The epidemic spread throughout the Balearic Isles like a brush fire. No one was immune to the hellish fever and accompanying symptoms. For many it was too late. Many wealthy displaced Europeans sought to flee any way they could. By private ferry, charter, in the smelly cargo hold of a trawler, boat yacht, . The butterfly effect in full swing. The pendulum in its never ending to and fro motion counted down the hours, minutes seconds…..to the next macabre never ending encore.

A couple savored a bottle of Bordeaux on board the sleek wooden hulled yacht moored in the bay near Marseilles. In the backdrop, the Chateau d'if, the notorious residence of thousands of political prisoners locked away inside the impenetrable fortress. As unescapable as Alcatraz. The setting for Alexander Dumas' Count of Monte Cristo.

They clinked their glasses savoring the still waters on the moonlit night. Not a soul in sight. They pledged their allegiance and undying love for one another. She was counting down the days to their 1st wedding anniversary. It had been a whirlwind round the world romance. Marseilles seemed like the perfect stop off point on the last leg of their tour, the final destination, the French Riviera. They decided to go for a dip. She peeled off her Angora sweater and leapt over the edge. He stumbled like a drunken sailor, smitten by her

love and tumbled overboard. She swam over to him to provide a little mouth to mouth.

"You didn't?!" she screamed. Forgetting to lower the ladder their only means of escape oft a fatal faux pas. And as it happened to all who sought to swim to shore after a valiant escape from Chateau d'If, No one ever reached the shore. Not one. A fin rose insidiously out of the water and beelined toward the boat. The two pairs of legs and arms dangling below the surface was too tempting to pass up. From their vantage point it appeared as only a sliver for a split second, an illusion, ere it was upon them.

"Meurdre" mumbled the mariner as he coughed up a bright red effluent as the great white literally tore them asunder. It's crazed albino eyes, evidence of harboring the fugitive, ebola once again offered a free ride, the victor in the vicious futile struggle.

If only they hadn't leapt over board, if only he'd lowered the ladder…if….the last fleeting thoughts that likely lingered in the minds of the star crossed lovers. In a few seconds all was silent. The tranquil waters of the bay were restored to their previous mirror sheen. The small erratically roving sets of razor sharp jaws continued to terrorize the endless miles of beaches from Barcelona to St Tropez. They left no catamaran or small dinghy unturned in their insatiable quest for food and a feeble attempt to end the madness that had crept into their craniums. The tiny unwanted visitor, the lethal virus ever present hitchin' a ride. It was not particular with regard to socioeconomic status or even species for that matter. As long as a rich source of blood supply presented itself, it could rapidly replicate and carry on indefinitely.

The 60 meter towering statue of Christopher Columbus peered over the Vell, or old harbor of Barcelona. The wise old sentinel kept a watchful eye on the massive marina. The perpetual motion of the swing bridge permitted passage to and fro into the inner sanctum. In the aligned position it also allowed the passage of droves of tourists and locals alike to visit the Mare Magnum, Europe's largest aquarium, 8000 fish including 11 sharks contained in 22 basins holding 1.5 million gallons of water. The small army of unwanted visitors, the outsiders, passed under the swing bridge seemingly unnoticed ever in search of their next meal.

Only the lone guardian, perched high atop the pedestal noticed. He soon had a few pesky preda-tors perch on his shoulders. Not the talkative parrots who accompanied him on the long sea voyage to the new land. But rather, the obnoxious black wing tipped bird of prey. Pharoah's vulture never ventured far from the silent partner in crime, the great white. The spoils were far too tempting. The birds waited patiently for the show was about to begin.

Several fisherman prepared for their fishing trips by emptying the bilges and storage com-partments in anticipation of a big catch of the day. They tossed the bloody bait overboard unaware of the silent intruder stalking the marina. The gentle-men were aghast as the large gaping orifice surf-aced and nearly joined them at the stern of the boat.

"Sacre bleu!"

"Le grand Blanc!" Au secour!"

Ere they reacted, the predator ripped an arm off the unwary seaman. Blood spurted all over the stern…sending a tantalizing aroma stirring the rest of the rabid sharks. A furious Frenchman moored only a few berths over responded. He'd lead the resistance, the charge of a light brigade of boats. Three loud blasts echoed over the marina as he backed the yacht from it's berth. The horn blasted as if to signal the vultures to 'come and get it.' The birds leapt from Columbus' shoulders and bore down on the bloody red pool swishing behind the captain with a vengeance. The bewildered boater aimed his flare gun at the flock, cackling loudly in a furious frenzy.

"Au revoir oiseaux!" he yelled defiantly and fired.

A fiery tail from the explosion shot across the marina and ignited the generous supply of alcohol fueling a cocktail party. It erupted in a loud fire-ball. The blast rocked the vessel and sent several guests overboard into the briny drink. Their arms flailed futilely. The startled crew sprung into action. They tossed a few life rings overboard yet ere they could scoop the social elite back on deck the hungry predators snatched them up. They disappeared without so much as an adieu. The predators greedily ground them to bite size pieces then came back for more. The vultures joined in the inviting soiree albeit the choice cuts had already disappeared. Nothing but slim pickens, skin and bones, They pecked relentlessly discarding the pearls, tiaras, rubies emeralds & expensive diamonds scattered about.

"Ouvre!" shouted the feisty Ahab like senior in hot pursuit. The crowd watched, stunned horror. Only a few able seamen joined the evening's festivities. The marine swing bridge operator was caught off guard unaware of the untimely incident. Ere he could respond and remotely activate the gentle swiveling motion of the bridge to let Ahab out, the swing bridge sheered the tall superstructure and one fuming fisherman from his perch. The upper deck, and seated seamen was hurled back into the enclosure. The sharks instantly veered in a violent u-turn to intercept the fishermen ere

he, his chair, and fishing rod sunk below the surface.

The shark's powerful jaws crushed the chair like a beer can and spit it out. Ahab like a slimy oyster slid down the gullet of the gaping hole.

Christopher watched the unfolding spectacle in silence from a safe distance. The blank expression of the statue stone cold fear. He could not imagine what fate awaited the new world as the vessels carried the ill, those on their death beds and the rotting putrid corpses toward the distant shores. The treacherous trek oft claimed the lives of many merchant mariners unawares. The cargo of gold and silver doubloon of immeasurable monetary value buried deep below the Atlantic. The USNS Comfort and Mercy beelined for Boston harbor with it's precious priceless cargo, victims. Many held the cure to the ebola conundrum, the key to a complete recovery locked inside their delicate DNA strands and blood yet to be decoded and unraveled. The ERs, waiting rooms, teams of doctors, nurses, EMTs, virologists, epidemiologists CDC and WHO experts eagerly awaited their arrival.

The smaller ill prepared clinics scattered through -out the Mediterranean fared far worse by the over- whelming surprise sneak attack. They began to fear a dreaded recurrence of a deadlier Spanish flu or influenza. Some sort of mutated bird flu….ebola hadn't even crossed many of the medical maven's minds until it was too late, accustomed to a few nasty gashes and broken bones, typical of the high seas fishing boats, sea sickness, the common cold …

Yet the indisputable death toll kept rising, surg- ing numbers, the cause of death - hemorrhagic fever, diarrhea, pain, bleeding did not forecast a promising prognosis.

The Ebola virus infected flocks of birds, vultures and sea creatures that swept across the Mediterranean in their relentless purge and culling spree. They crept ever closer toward Naples, to mete out vengeance on the US naval base like ISIS or Al Qaeda terrorists. Sardinia and Corsica stood in the way. Not even the notorious well armed Cosa Nostra nor shepherds tending their herds of goats on the gentle slopes could contain the tiny deceptive u shaped shepherd's crook contagion. All cloaked inside an unwary ever shape changing host, mammal, bird or fish, no matter, oft going about their daily routine, eating and flying to their next port.

Porto Cervo was one such locale. The secluded sleepy seaside playground and haunt of the rich was a far cry from the impoverished villages all along the coast. Some of the most coveted caviar, finest wines and exclusive cuts of lamb, and tempting seafood offered so generously by the not so well off neighbors. No matter ebola and its host proved an equal opportunity opportunistic sampler of hospitality.

A young couple had spent a week in the lap of luxury at one of the most exclusive retreats in the world. The Cala Di Volpi hotel amongst a handful at the top of the charts. The airy decadent rooms opened to an unforgettable vista near the quaint 'Deer's port', or Porto Cervo. Home to billionaire playboys and well heeled partiers.

The temptress toyed with her stilettos. She reached across the bed and filled the contoured footwear and extended it to her male companion.

"Like leading a horse to the trough" she giggled. Her Italian stallion bowed his head eagerly in her never ending enticing games. Their vicarious charades carried on well into the wee hours of the morn. She'd oft tip toe from her private deck opening onto a breathtaking vista near the marina. Then slip aboard her boyfriend's sleek yacht and start all over again.

"Let the games begin." The debutante's acrobatic antics drove her debonair industrialist wild. She oft boasted about how flexible and limber she was. He responded by eating the caviar from her exposed belly button as she willingly arched her back. On the spacious deck. Then cartwheel with a resound-ing splash in the crystal clear waters of either the onboard pool or the marina. The choice was always clearly hers. And today unlike any other, the speedo clad stud savored every moment as he noshed the roe from the tiny receptacle in her
mid section.

"Stop that, it tickles" she giggled, from her

viewpoint, the world upside down, topsy turvy, head over heels in love. "Now watch this" she commanded. He washed the delectable roe down with a splash of the finest Rothchild.

She dizzily reached for the deck, head over heels she negotiated several cartwheels, feeling frisky she avoided the wading pool and leapt off the end of the streamlined vessel. Ere she hit the water a great white broadsided her like a deer in a jeep's headlights. The impact snapped her in two like a twig. The two halves of her bloody entrails quickly snatched up by the accompanying blood thirsty predators.

"Ciao bella" said her absent minded suitor as he hurried to answer an important call inside the main cabin.

When he returned his temptress was nowhere

to be found. He loved how she teased him. A challenging game of hide and seek amongst the staterooms and numerous decks. Always arousing, taunting…

As he stepped down onto the platform almost flush with the water, he bent down to examine the bloody red film floating on the water. He feared one of the other yacht owners may soon face a pricey overhaul of the massive transmission driving the behemoth. He rubbed the liquid in his fingers. It was not oily or slippery.

Before the Italian stallion could turn his head toward the loud thud, he was broadsided by the massive marine monster. It's jaws agape, not the agape love he'd felt for his fiancé. There was no love lost as the predator slid across the wooden deck and disappeared on the opposite side. The level headed crooner reached out as his life flashed before his eyes. In a futile desperate attempt, he grabbed a spear gun leaning on the edge. As the jaws closed and sealed his fate, a loud snap, the crunching of bone severed his arm which dropped lifelessly onto the deck, the spear gun still firmly locked in his grip. It would be some time before any of the neighbors bothered to board, to begin their usual night time antics. Ebola waited, with baited breath. It would soon find a new host, oblivious of their well heeled upbringing. The harbinger of doom had successfully landed on every isle in the Mediterranean to carry out it's inevitable mission. Eventually every body of water, lake, inlet to wipe every living creature off the map in it's ever expanding quest to survive. . It had nearly encompassed the western Mediterra-nean. Was there no deterrent to match the deadly firepower of this elusive entity?

6: Pino(t)cchio?

"Thou tellest my wanderings;
put thou my tears in thy bottle;
are they not in thy book?"

- Psalm 56:8 KJV

The descent proved much more difficult than the ascent, the delicate contents of her back pack slowing her down, now her main priority. The goal was to reach the distant foot of the rich fertile lava gouged slopes of Mount Vesuvius in once piece. It seemed like an eternity. Katherine's eyes stung in the hot noon day sun. She found little comfort in the fact that she'd soon indulge herself in the lap of luxury in the quaint enticing hotel ensuite. A fine black mist of lava dust rose then dissipated with each weary belabored step. The painful irritating scratching in her corneas was unbearable. She closed her eyes and dreamt of the cascading waterfall awaiting her. The powerful placebo provided little relief. She trudged on tormented by the pin pricks pushing into her eye sockets. At last, sweet victory was theirs as the tired team entered the outskirts of Naples at the base of the tempera-mental peak that had blown it's top back in 69 AD. The weary souls sauntered toward the airy patio terrace. A collection of sorts were savoring the fruits of their labors. Upon closer examination, they seemed an odd couple, one local seasoned connoisseur and a tourist, perhaps a travel or parasitic food and wine writer dabbling in the delectable delights the region had to offer. The laughter overflowed as did the offering of the gods.

"Pass the pinot" slurred the tourist. The elder patron reached for an amber colored bottle of Vin Santo or "holy wine" from amongst the colorful rainbow and generously filled the half full glass.

"Ahhh, would you not agree I saved the best for last?"

"Indeed."

"Mind if we join you?" asked the bodacious albeit battered and bruised lone female. "Our palettes and eyes are parched whilst our egos are bruised."

"Please do sit down. This is just what the doctor ordered."

"Graci." She sipped the sweet nectar of the gods slowly, a potent pinot blanc which imme-diately tickled her nasal cavity. She blushed and blinked relentlessly as the spirits raced to her head. "Ahh, a beautiful bouquet" she babbled.

"Perhaps the lady would prefer the rose known as Occhio de Pernice or Eye of the Partridge?" With a keen eye, he'd noticed her peculiar predicament.

"You share the same passion our savior once displayed as the devil was cast from heaven."

"Excuse me?"

"Diablo was expelled much to the delight of Il Figlio de Dio. Gesu Christo was so ecstatic he erupted in tears of joy."

Katherine regained her composure. With an air of skepticism she scoffed at the old geezer.

"That's a good one Geppetto."

He shrugged his shoulders oblivious to the connotation.

"Geppetto & Pinocchio?" added his adroit side kick.

The senior emitted a hearty chuckle that spread to his belly like a bowlful of jelly.

"Si Consuella."

"My name's Katherine."

"He's not kidding. Swear to God" insisted the sidekick as his eyes roamed skyward.

"The flood of emotion bathed the deeply scarred landscape from past lava flows. A rich fertile soil resulted whilst divine inspiration did the rest. The vineyards are amongst the region's finest."

Katherine cast another skeptical glance at the geriatric geezer.

"Cross my heart, hope to die if I tell a lie." His weary weather beaten severely bent digits bore the mark of a veteran vintner as he raised them slowly toward his chest. He then cast a glance beyond the summit of Vesuvius and thanked God. "Graci."

"So he's not some two bit hocus pokus Pinocchio peddler?

"No ma'am, he isn't. But you might say he does know his 'Pinotcchio', Pinot as in wine and Occhio as in eyes."

"The eyes have it" he concurred.

"I'm sorry I don't follow this bubbly psycho babble."

"Let me have a look" as he stood up and

sauntered toward her. He studied her grief stricken grimace and delicately raised a set of glasses to his saddle bag laden eyes. The comical Magoo like character ogled her and offered her some hope.

"Are you done?"

"Yes, miss. May I offer you some advice?"

"I know I could use a little mascara, but it bothers my eyes unbearably."

"I know." He sat down and wrote something illegibly on a wrinkled napkin. "Force of habit." He shoved the napkin toward her.

"What's up doc? Isn't it time they took you back home, uh the senior's home is it?"

"Ha, ha, ha" he chuckled.

"Doc Oc here may have just what the doctor ordered. Oc uh Occhio or eye as in Opthalmology one of the noted authorities on eye diseases in Italy. His son followed in his footsteps. Fortunately as fate would have it, in a rather odd serendipitous series of events you stumbled upon…"

"I'm so sorry." Yet no tears of joy welled up in her dry eyes.

"No need to apologize. My son, Dr Mancini, 'branched out' you might say and embarked on a voyage."

"One can't discover a new land until one loses sight of the shore" she said bleary eyed.

"He soon discovered a new exciting emerging field - regenerative medicine right here under our noses at the world's oldest state university.

"Good old Napoli U."

"Replacing limbs and the like?"

"Yes. With one's own cells, stem cells."

"Who knew?" Katherine sat in awe as Doc Oc revealed the secrets of science like a sacred geriatric guru. A bulbous buddha or prophet planted amongst his pinots and 'holy wine'.

"Ah here we are. Well bon appetite."

The chef had prepared the finest angus steak tartar topped with the precious yellow yolk from the brown eggs Katherine herself had plucked from the slopes of Vesuvius. The rare specimens of Canary Egyptian Vulture eggs. Well beyond the boundaries of their usual expansive migratory pattern. It was a rare treat indeed. Katherine poked the membrane, as thin as a contact lens, covering the yellow liquid as precious as gold in some parts. It spilled it's contents like an over flowing reservoir onto the porous meaty perimeter…the irresistible combination to die for.

"A toast, to friends, family and a bright happy future" motioned Magoo then downed the savory sweet nectar, a gift from Go's only begotten son and a handful of the finest vintners this side of Naples..

"Down the hatch." Katherine placed the savory sumptuous liquid laced meat onto her tongue. It tasted divine, and slid down her throat to her stomach very smoothly. It mingled with the digestive juices and was soon absorbed into her circulatory system for the short trip straight to the heart. Unwittingly they had all unleashed the harbinger of doom, like a toxic, lethal injection, it was only a matter of time, a couple of days at most, before the deadly effects would reveal themselves. They devoured the decadent serving and begged for more. Each guest had now consumed a lethal dose of Ebola. The real question was, how long would their deaths go unnoticed? How was the local population to react to their untimely sudden deaths? How would the local authorities treat and deal with such an insidious disaster, possibly a national pandemic.

"There's plenty more where that came from" mentioned Magoo, the gracious host hoped to satisfy their unquenchable hunger and thirst.

A group of navy seals training offshore from the US naval base in Naples noticed the unusual behavior of the predator. The crazed killing machine converged on the helpless couple thrashing

about in the water next to their overturned catamaran.

"We're not gonna make it!" shouted the SAR team leader.

The insatiable appetite of the ebola virus mean-dering about within the gyrations and gullies of the shark's grey matter had literally created a monster. Out of it's mind, it slipped out of sight then bee-lined for the both of the bewildered boaters. The creature latched onto their legs above the knees then pulled them under in a violent dance of death. The sea turned a bright red ere the rescuers could react.

The zodiac approached the scene of the gruesome crime cautiously, the eagle eyes scoured the water for any and all signs of life.

All they could drag from the bloody sea was a stained life preserver and a sailor's hat. The seals had sealed their own fate unknowingly. Ebola had come all the way up the food chain, care of the largest cruise liner and the great whites. The spoiled fish had followed the 6th fleet all the way back to the base in Naples on their spread of anarchy and carnage all along Mediterranean. From the sunny shores of Majorca to the south of France. From the pristine beaches frequented by Parisians along the French Riviera and St Tropez. The enraged ebola laiden eating machines sought to slay everything it their path in their vicious never ending cycle.

"We're gonna need some back up" shouted a seal nervously ere the catamaran keeled over. The seals swung a sharp hairpin u turn and roared for the destroyer. The medic applied a cold compress as they prepared to pass him off to the waiting unwary crew. Ebola was allowed to slip in under the radar like a stow away, or implanted spy.

"You got it Pontiac" shouted the base commander of the secure naval computer and telecommunications station. Their worst nightmare had resurfaced as he peered at the pinterest like map of the Mediterranean. Not to depict the chief's favorite beaches to check out in his impending shore leave albeit the red dots did map out a clearly obvious pattern of attack. The usual breeding grounds in the migratory pattern of the marine menace. It was clear that ebola's host had created several beach heads from which the invader could certainly strike fast and furious. Reports of shark attacks flooded the airwaves. The trendy tourist haunts rendered speechless, their spirits dampened, now mere ghost towns. Coupled with countless shark attacks and the EVD - Ebola Virus Disease scare, it took its toll. The world class eateries and resorts vacated. To add insult to injury, several clinics along the coast continued to be overwhelmed by a series of similar flu like symptoms. Fatigue, dizziness, pain, chills and bloody expulsions spilling all over the ERs. Most of the victims succumbed to a horrible tragic end in a matter of days.

"How could we be so blind?" The commander slapped his forehead in disgust. "I'm afraid the admiral will be forced to wipe the egg off his face in a futile attempt to eat his own words."

"This son of a b 's come back with a vengeance!"

"What the f….lorence nightingale?" the lady with the lamp, a harbinger of hope while tending the troops during the Crimean War. The admiral's vocal volcanic eruption abruptly shattered the gala seaside dinner gathering. The soothing sounds and soft lantern lighting encircling the compound , a dramatic backdrop against Mt Vesuvius in the distance ceased.

"I hate to be the one, but I told you so" did not begin to sum up the ruined admiral's intuition and reputation let alone his arrogant brash and brazen proclamation a mere month ago. 'Mission Accom-plished'...the words resonated in his mind now revving a mile a minute. How had he let this eva-sive entity slip though his fingertips. Like an insidious Al Qaeda or ISIS insurgence, about to knock on his very back door and join the festivi-ties, in his own bloody back yard for God's sakes. It was too much to swallow. A shockwave surged up and down his left arm. He reached for a glass of house wine, none other than the revered Lacryma Christi, Home grown right here on fertile slopes of Naples. His bleary eyes failed to focus as he tipped the contents of the glass. The dark red liquid dissi-pated quickly soaking up to the edge of the white table cloth. The distinguished list of dignitaries and former naval commanders weren't amused. The admiral, known for his sordid tall tales, loud and boisterous outbursts thought him par for the course.

"That reminds me, will you be joining our foursome , Hank, at 7 am sharp?"

"Why of course" said the admiral confidently as he regained his composure. He'd received 'good tidings' like this countless times before. He was certainly up for the challenge. Word travelled through the naval command center at the speed of thought. Specialized task forces were briefed about what they were potentially up against. The enemy unlike all the rag tag rebels and ill equipped soldiers of the past, was keen, cunning. Inspite of the entity's tiny size, relatively unprotected body, essentially unarmed, it packed quite a punch. The medical personnel could not harp enough on the gravity of the situation enough. Like the magic DU, depleted uranium, bullets they'd used to blast through armor, to plant the seeds of destruction on an unsuspecting enemy. The shoe or army boot now squarely on the other foot, the tables drama-tically turned as the soldiers prepared for combat. The arms race had ramped up to a veritable space race against an alien like invasion. Soldiers donned hermetically sealed gas masks, a grim, ghostly reminder of an updated version their fore fathers wore waging a deadly hand to hand combat in the mustard gas infiltrated trenches. A subtle change in wind direction could wipe out an entire battalion. They'd fare no better against this elusive entity that could change its shape then resurface anywhere anytime, at random, oft behind enemy lines or even nip them in the bud. The admiral checked his busy schedule. Ironically an upcoming operetta, 'Naple's Soldier' by the renown Andrea Bocelli, only a fortnight away. First sung during the Spanish influenza of 1918 which left some half a billion dead he recalled. The eerie translation struck a chord, - 'Naple's Soldier', the most popular tune might be as catchy as the Spanish flu or ebola virus. He scratched out the scribbled notes in his daily ledger. Appointments, special speak-ing engagements, appearances, paying princely sums to novices lapping up his expertise and illustrious career accomplishments. Page upon page ripped out, the final chapter left blank. He'd reserved an indefinite period of time to put an end to this threat once and for all.

The cargo hold was crammed with frightened, famished, fish out of water. The dark cramped hold held almost a thousand migrant workers eager to begin a new life in Italy. The treacherous trek through the Aegean Sea between Greece and Turkey tossed the vessel too and fro. As if reliving famous battles of Troy or Sparta, fortunately they'd been spared their lives. Many had given their life savings, some resorted to stealing and petty crime just to scrape together the $5000 dollars to pay the nefarious ferrymen. They herded the sizeable load aboard, reaping a clean $3.5 million profit quickly dispersed amongst the rag tag pirates.

"We'll start afresh, a new leaf. Believe me, it will work out" stated the talented Turk. A skilled craftsmen and goat herder. He'd sold his paintings for pennies, merely to trade in exchange for future fortunes. His wife smiled convinced they'd made the right decision. They were filled with hope. As the ship neared the distant shore as if coming to America, their hearts skipped a beat at the beautiful coastline.

"Land!"

The parched passengers, packed like lemmings sought relief from their confines. They could not stand the stale air and putrid stench of feces and urine any more. The armed guard overwhelmed by the mob, was shoved aside in the ensuing stampede

He relinquished his weapon ere the other thugs could react. Gambling away the proceeds of their carefully concocted human trafficking scam.

"Vesuvius…it's more beautiful than the post-cards", even one of the paintings that procured his trip proclaimed the proud Turk. He grabbed his wife and placed her on his shoulders so she could get a better look. The mad mob fought frantically clamoring to get up top, on the deck.

"Stop them!" shouted the ring leader. They let off several rounds into the air… but the over-whelming surge of stifled human slaves pushed forth.

"If you shut up truth and bury it under the ground it will but grow, and gather such explosive power that the day it bursts through it will blow up every-thing in it's way!" shouted the wise Turk citing Emile Zola's immortal words. The top heavy cargo vessel rocked uncontrollably inspite of the traffick-ers futile attempts to contain the crowd. It toppled, overturned and in an instant compressed a mass of mystified mariners in the sinking steel coffin. Their curiosity coupled with the sheer weight had sealed their fate. No one escaped…as the ship sunk to the bottom of the bay of Naples. Not even the valiant efforts of the navy seals and countless seaman who raced to the horrific scene could save them. The only signs of life were two of the traffickers still toting their AK 47's defiantly high in the air. All to no avail. The seals rounded them up, lassoed them in less than eight seconds and herded them off to await their fate. Their days of endless round trips, rounding up and herding the most vulnerable, gullible foreigners oft marked by greed, deception and ultimately death, were over. The transfers took a terrible toll, torn families, shattered dreams in a last ditch effort to flee their misfortunes only to die on foreign soil or at sea. A vicious cycle, the cycle of life continued. The sole victors in this tragedy, the countless carnivorous cartilage-nous killers, crunching on the contents of the cargo hold like a humungous can of tuna or sardines. The uncanny carnage marked by short lived screams subsided as many succumbed to the salt water filling their lungs. The predators penetrated the periphery for a free for all inside. Inside the hosts lurked a far greater insidious entity. Ebola merely transferred or passed along like a pawn on the giant watery playing field. A third party, the ever present birds of prey con-verged on the feisty few who had surfaced, only to have their entire body bombarded by the relentless pecking. Phar-oah's chicken, the Canary vulture, ISIS chosen spread it's wings in flight to proli-ferate and spread it's seeds of destruction far and wide. The next move undoubtedly up to the admiral. The fate of man-kind may very well rest in his trusted hands. He had a golden opportunity to end this repetitive naval nonsense once and for all.

“That’s the last of the lot” said the seaman on the verge of vomiting. He had never witnessed such disregard for human life. Instead of new found freedom, their last gruesome moments spent in utter terror awaiting a grizzly death.

The bodies were placed in the endless array of body bags set up in the makeshift morgue near the naval base slated for incineration. Not only had ebola defiantly defeated every attempt to contain it, it now landed on the front door steps of the admir-alty and staff waiting to be welcomed with open arms like a newborn into the family.

7: On The Rocks

"Sometimes by losing a battle you find a new way to win the war."

- Donald Trump, billionaire, entrepreneur, presidential candidate

The epidemic had spread as far as the eastern extremity of the Mediterranean. It left no stone unturned like ISIS carnivorous chosen, the ornery vultures laid their eggs everywhere to insure its continued lineage. Every nook and remote cranny, over hill and dale, and yonder glen. Pharoah's chicken was seemingly coming home to roost and face a final showdown? An avian aerial Armageddon. An airborne assault the likes of which the world had never seen before? Were we all just sitting ducks waiting for the final curtain call? The onus was on us, mankind, to take the bull or the devil by the horns and send him back to where he belonged.

"I have this uneasy queasy feeling in the pit of my stomach" said the beautiful blonde bombshell lapping it all up in the luxurious Aphrodite Hill Spa named the number one in all of Europe.

The trained fingers of the therapist tenderly an-nointed the ravishing guest with virgin olive oil, emollients and a select blend of floral extracts. The herbal cleanse massaged into every pore, protuberance and orifice. The nervousness from within eventually gave way to a state of ecstatic elation bordering on orgasm. She hadn't felt this alive in ages. Like a rebirth, Rebecca had been given a new lease on life thanks to the kind hearted, generous gentleman waiting for her in the pool. The exclusive spa nestled in the hills provided a breath taking perspective of the port of Paphos and the enchanting Cyprus coastline.

After their invigorating workout, her suitor convinced her to accompany him to the most romantic spot, his favorite in the entire world. He urged her to close her eyes, then tied the silky smooth mat-erial around her head. Pitch black, bound, she was now at the mercy of this man. A tingling sensation

surged through her body magnified by the massage that morning. The noon day sun beat down on them as he led her over the hot sand. She hopped like a bunny over the tingling white sand.

"Just a few more steps." The anticipation was killing her. Her set her gently against the smooth weather beaten surface and tied the silky wrap around her. "Open them." He withdrew the blindfold. Rebecca squinted then blinked a few times. The breathtaking panorama coupled with a kiss unnerved her. He pressed his lips against hers. He'd never let her go.

"Where, pray tell are we?"

"The place where the most beautiful woman on earth was born."

"You mean to tell me I'm not the most ravishing creature you've ever laid your eyes on?" she quipped facetiously.

"You are equal in every way, my fair Aphrodite."

"Walk this way" she said enticingly.

"Legend has it Aphrodite was born on this

very spot. As the sea surged, a white foam enveloped the rock named after her. Anyone who swims around it will be blessed with eternal beauty."

"What are we waiting for?"

She tossed the silky red fabric into the air then dashed into the crystal clear waters. "race yuh" she yelled ecstatically.

The red ribbon was swept out to sea. It soon snagged on what appeared to be floating debris …the rising hump alarmed him. Like a matador's cape caught in the horns of a feisty fuming, charging bull, the fabric caught the front edge of the large pointy fin. The red tail fluttered in the sea breeze as the predator gained speed past the rock. A few wide eyed vultures had perched atop the rock. Front row seats to the spectacle like Romans at the Coliseum, then as if to signal thumbs down they flocked off…to sort through the scraps. He was numb. Petrified, stone cold fear embraced him. His beloved, so close, yet so far away. He could never reach her in time, but he had to try. Roman waved his arms in the air frantically. He dove into the water to beeline toward her. Rebecca waved back….as the menacing monster dove beneath the surface, and left his calling card. The red marker as if to say 'I was here' or x marks the spot. Such a bizarre bewildering ending thought Roman. Rebecca disappeared beneath the thunderous surging red swell... totally consumed in the moment. The persistent predators were the undisputed victors once again as their swath of carnage and ruthless killing spree continued. More feared than ISIS, or any prior evil epidemic. The impending global pandemic was gaining ground. It's maniacal spread across all borders by leaps and bounds knowing not when or how to stop. No end in sight to the vicious vicarious viral mayhem.

In a short time the great white and the accompanying aerial freeloaders found their way to Tel Aviv. Founded on the rocky outcrop at Jaffa, the historical treasure trove dating back to before the time of Christ had transformed into a coveted high tech trading capital of the world.

The great white ventured into the warm inviting waters off the picturesque promenade in Jaffa meaning beautiful or beauty in Hebrew. Ironically near the very spot where Jonah met his match and spent the better part of three days in the belly of the beast. This formidable foe had no intention of ceding its captives nor coughing them up in a couple of days. Its perpetual motion, driven in order to survive and thrive coupled with an insatiable hunger scanned his prospects. The seawall rebuilt after the great flood in Noah's day had withstood the test of time. Legend had it that Andromeda was tied to it naked awaiting her fate. Perseus slew several notorious nemesis and sea monsters, a Gorgon Medusa and Cetus the whale ere her rescued her. None as bold or brash and brazen dared to enter the shark infested waters. A Super Dvora III patrol boat was dispatched by the Israeli navy. With its thrust vectoring like the F35 II Lightning, it zigged and zagged around slower yachts and vessels as it raced to the scene at more than 50 knots. The fast and furious response was no match for the ruthless predator. He sought to satiate his hunger and nosh on a few new arrivals dashing to the water's edge. Oblivious to the foreboding menace off shore, they dove in head over heels.

The aerial invasion accompanied the naval assault. Pharoah's chicken managed several fly-by's anxiously awaiting the fate of the daring sea divers. The Super D arrived in the nick of time and unleashed a stream of rapid fire lead into the air. The iron dome like defenses, bombs bursting in the air, plucked the plentiful plumage to the bone. The wily eyed vultures fell from the sky in the firestorm. The menacing toothy man eater met his fate shortly thereafter from a precisely guided AGM hellfire surface to surface missile. It found the target, one gaping hole, and oversized stuffed gullet. The predator was strewn all over the promenade, the red entrails sprayed the sea wall like modern art deco graffiti. It served as a reminder and stern warning to all who dared to disrupt the peace and prosperity of the port, to think twice!

Two Dabur patrol boats tagged along and arrived

fashionably late, just in case, to clean up the scraps. They admired the fancy artwork on the wall. Like red rolling hills awash, a wavy line steeped in the cascading red droplets. Depicting the fall of communism, fascism - the Berlin Wall and all other futile attempts to segregate people with protective concrete enclosures like the Palestine Wall, or proposed Mexico Wall like mindless sheep. Separate rabbits by an endless fence in Australia only to have them burrow beneath the surface and continue to procreate at will on either side.

The carnage had spread across the entire Mediterranean. The circle complete. The noose tightened, everything inside it's perimeter permanently irreversibly infected, destined to die a horrible painful death.

Was there no escape from this hellish recurring nightmare? The virologists fought feverishly trying to up the antidotes available but the labs lagged far behind. Experimental vaccines were brought out of frozen storage, locked vaults, compromised military protocol in a futile attempt to battle this insidious foe. More fearsome than any previous Ebola outbreak, or Influenza epidemic. It struck with a vengeance without rhyme or reason like Al Qaeda, ISIS , or Taliban terrorist attack. But it's ever widening circle of carnage was inevitably destined to grow.

From sea to decimated sea, the Mediterranean lay in ruin. Casualties rose rapidly on every remote rock, isle and resort. The virus overran resources, resilient resourceful attempts by medics and first responders. Lines were drawn in the sand. Heroic battles were valiantly fought. But the beast emer-ged with a vengeance more determined than ever. The ticking time bomb that scientists had warned us about, and harped on for so long, had not been heeded. Mankind's worst fears had come to fruition. The ever changing form of the virus as it jumped from host to host, species to species was unimaginable.

St Bernard's upgraded façade and facilities in the solitary outpost in Europort to oversee the British territory at the foot of the Rock of Gibraltar was slated to open it's doors. From the 60 million pound injection, the modern facility had swelled to three times it's size. Designed to handle surgery, ortho, hydrotherapy, maternity, trauma and hydrotherapy. 210+ beds were completely swamped. A small dose of drugs had arrived a fortnight ago. The injured had arrived in EMT ambulances, cars, taxis, shopping carts. Eager Europeans hoped to cash in on the free health care. It taxed the system immeasurably. The strain and extra long shifts endured by the ER staff took it's toll. They were on the brink, coffers depleted, the medical supplies desperately low, when the inconceivable occurred. A rare downpour, of torrential magnitude, accompanied by thunderous lightning disrupted the electricity to much of the city of 30,000. Several transformers were knocked out after violent sequential explosions. The backup generators sputtered, some kicked in, some emitted a dark plume of smoke having sat idle likely since the dark ages. The double whammy was all that most of the tense staff needed to send them over the top, into a tailspin. Tensions rose, some snapped, either literally or figurative with inflamed flowery outbursts.

A world away, three civilized savages sought an answer to their dilemma. How to transfer a boat-load of beautiful begonias or petunias as Emma had so comically mislabeled them.

"Hit me again" she requested, to refresh her delightful virgin cocktail.

"Only this time, make it … straight up… … on the rocks."

Barry complied hesitantly. His thoughts drifted to his joint venture, a million miles away from the maddening crowd or congested streets of Madagascar. The reason he had sought shelter off shore in the secluded sanctity of the Seychelles. Their banking system virtually bulletproof and at more than arm's length of the law.

"Out of sight, out of mind" he quipped. Grateful to have always gone the extra mile, literally to get away from the prying bureaucratic eyes of the buffoons and his lack luster lackadaisical colleagues.

"They missed the boat, the mark completely,. They'll never leave a legacy" he fumed.

"Easy does it on the coconut juice chief" quipped Bernie. He'd oft saved the party ere they departed as lost souls or OD. Boasting of an acquired taste to a Bloody Mary when in fact it was laced with a half a bottle of Tabasco. He feared Emma may face a similar unwelcome upheaval.

"I'm just sayin'."

"All's well that ends well" offered Bernie. But Barry sunk into the captain's seat of his aging fishing boat.

"Is that all there is?"

"You mean if all roads leads to Rome? Let 'em have it. Besides, look what happened to Rome."

"Caligula, carnage, copulation, complete and utter corruption, ultimately collapse...."

"That's quite a mouthful."

"Must be the meds and coconuts talking" as she grabbed her melons and adjusted her bikini top not acclimatized to the sweltering heat yet.

"I'll take USey, a little grass shack by the beach, a blonde bombshell and a bottle of gin any day."

Emma seemed delirious. Combining even trace amounts of alcohol with the deadly anti cancer / Ebola concoction could be fatal, definitely not what either doctor ordered.

Barry eyed the ever present predator drones buzzing about, roaming the port. A strong US presence necessary to patrol the deadly waters all the way up the coast past Kenya, primarily into Somalia.

"Seychelles may be out of sight of the Horn of Africa, a whole host of Somali pirates and Yemeni terrorist training camps but.... They're always lurking.... in the back of my mind."

"At least it keeps the natives from getting a little restless."

Emma fell into a much needed deep sleep mumbling the words of the great F. Scott:

"Doctor (Oncology) is the best
Sends no bills and takes no rest
Brings to pain and broken bone
Pharmacopeia all it's own.
His assistant Dr Bed
Likes to coddle me instead
Soothes me in his private room
Recreates the healthy womb.

Meet the jolliest of the three

My psychiatrist Dr B

Dear old bottle slaps my back

When I'm just about to crack.'"

The laptop erupted in an erratic state of confusion. The overwhelming hustle and bustle of the swamped ER or OR caught the two medical mavens both unawares.

"We're up to our eyeballs in Ebola" screamed his colleague, the silent partner in their shell company and joint venture from St Bernard's Hospital. The recipient of the generous UGib grant was only seed capital, the tip of the iceberg. What they needed was a massive injection if they were to nip this virus in the bud. "It's now or never. We need more of the CEV 7 vaccine."

He hung onto every syllable as the image transformed into a fuzzy blur. The signal lost likely to the ill timed power outage and an online disruption of service.

"We're in deep shit!"

"Nothing these sea worthy tankers can't tackle."

"Ebola 'll be tasting a croissant in a patisserie in Paris, sipping a fine wine down the Rhine or crossing the channel and having tea with her highness or haunting an enchanted Scottish castle ere we ever got there."

Barry pulled back on the frame of a fake Gaugin.

"Sweet."

He fumbled with the combination of the safe.

"Trains, seaplanes or automobiles won't get us there on time." He grabbed the small black box.

"Let me guess. Pandora's Box?" said Bernie facetiously.

"It's our only hope."

He opened the padded compartment. It looked like a chemistry set either of them might've opened on Christmas Day decades ago; inspiring one

to an illustrious career as a Chemist or Oncologist. "My private stash. I've been saving this for a rainy day." Countless foamy compartments stuffed with the vital vials. The fruits of his labors. Over a decade of trials and errors, hits and misses. He felt he had a home run. A viable vaccine. Emma, the missing piece of the puzzle. Her bloodwork had confirmed their suspicions. The lingering question burning in their minds was where did Will get it? From military storage? From a notorious network of tinkering scientists like themselves? Or far worse the black market. The elusive 'which came first the chicken or egg?' conundrum. Why only one syringe? Overkill to say the least, one syringe could treat a thousand patients. Why only Emma? Was it meant for her use only? Did he not have time to explain to her? Did he not know? Perhaps he placed so little trust in the vaccine? Likely obtained from the black market. Sheer suicide? Someone seemed to have placed little faith in their endeavor.

8: Eye in the Sky

"The sky is the daily bread of the eyes."

- Ralph Waldo Emmerson

A long line of feeble limbed, blinded, maimed well after the endless strife, the result of millions of buried land mines abandoned after civil wars. They held onto each other's hands like a conga line or barrel of monkeys. They had crossed countless miles of rain forest and a border to get here. Many of the fortunate ones wore a patch only over one eye. The rest were completely blind either from birth or from the devastating scourge of the latest ebola outbreak. The patient nurse, herded her little enthusiastic entourage toward the end of the dusty unmarked runway. The majority of connect-ing hubs and smaller airports had already closed in a last ditch effort by authorities from spreading the virus, now suspected of exhibiting airborne prop-erties.

They anxiously awaited the familiar loud prop-eller driven sounds of the smaller humanitarian smuggling efforts. Medical supplies, basic food stuffs and dried goods, precious water. The contraband oft swiped from the contaminated shelves of other infected hospitals and remote outposts. The pathetic cycle of poverty and hand me downs never ended. Yet they were all glad and blessed just to be alive to spend even one more day on this earth. The faithful flock was startled by the strange sound of the turbine engines as the McDonnell Douglas DC 10 touched down . The mighty roar of the mighty twin engines that hung from each wing rang out over the jungle. The pilots slammed on the brakes, and pushed the reverse thrusters hard to come to a stop on the short run-way.

"We're not gonna make it!" shouted the pilot.

"By the grace of God!"

"You're not turning religious on me are you?"

"Look up ahead."

Countless tiny arms flew up into the air. They waved them feverishly. The nurse noticed the plane barreling down the runway. It was quickly running out of real estate.

"Come on!" she yelled….She tugged their tiny hands. "Get out of the way!"

The children's smiles did not turn to sheer terror as the menacing roar was almost upon them. Many were completely blind.

As faith or dumb blind luck would have it, the large wheels which could've crushed them, rolled on by. The pilots bowed their head in prayer, sweating bullets.

As soon as the screams of joy burst into the air, and the smiling faces appeared on the cockpit windows, it laid the pilots' worst fears to rest.

The crew greeted the afflicted entourage with open arms. Defying orders to avoid direct contact with contaminated children and adults, the pilots hugged the happy go lucky tots and held them in their arms.

The medical doctor shook his head still donning a mask and goggles. He looked like an overgrown minion. Fearing he'd soon have to treat his pilots and ground crew, he hurried the pediatric patients aboard. Special precautions were taken to treat them. The operatory and recovery rooms were covered in layers of hermetically sealed drapes. The microscopes and surgical lasers were equally protected.

"Welcome aboard the 'flying eye hospital'."

The kids rushed aboard the large strange aircraft feeling their way along the hospital's side corridor. The children were seated in the modern classroom situated behind the cockpit. Unlike any other one room school house the few that had any sight at all could recall. Their tiny legs, too short to touch the colorful caret, swayed to and fro in a timely beat.

One by one the doctor examined them. He instructed them to open their eyes as the nurse gently lifted the patch from either eye, in some cases both.

"Let me have a look at you" said the ophthalmologist. He could've been an astronaut in some sort of space suit as far as the children were concerned. They had never seen either professional. It was overwhelming, all so frightening and new.

"My God. I've never seen so many affected irises and corneas". He shined the bright opthalmoscope into each eye. It exhibited the characteristic signs of the presence of the ebola virus. Presumably only one eye. He was shocked to discover so many victims that harbored the virus in both eyes. A bizarre collection of multicolored irises and corneas presented themselves. ‘

“It’s a sign” suggested the nurse, sitting on both sides of the fence, science based yet brought up religious. ”of the times. End times.”

“Every African country we’ve touched down in.” Orbis had orbited the dark continent like a spying CIA satellite. The big eye in the sky had made several flybys round the clock in a never ending cycle. The fuel, let alone the plane, generously supplied by Fedex. Oft smuggled in under cover of the night in old 45 gallon drums discarded by dictators.

“I’m surprised we ever got off the ground in Ghana.”

Several close calls, escaping by the skin of their teeth, far too close for comfort.

The child was prepped for a quick 'pin prick' like poking a hole in an egg, then a pop, pop, fizz, fizz. "Oh what a relief it is" as the delicate procedure to extract the essence of the evil, the Ebola virus from within the victim's eyeball. The contaminated elixir was squirted into a safely sealed canister to be discarded at their earliest convenience. Usually incinerated in a small service near the runway right after the last surgery. To prevent the possibility of spreading the virus and in the remote likelihood of theft or a rebel ramsacking. "Knock on wood" said the ophthalmologist as the nurse wiped the beads of sweat from his eyes.

The children were put to rest in the recovery

room. The nurse added a small prayer of gratitude for each and every one of them.

"Give us this day our daily bread and forgive us our trespasses as we forgive those who trespass against us. Shhh!" she urged the children. The sound of distant gunfire crept ever closer. Her eyes darted around the room. Even with their restored sight, fleeing into the forest meant certain death. Easy prey for the gorillas or the guerillas. Either way they were as good as dead. She continued to whisper to the very end. "For thine is the power, the kingdom and the glory, forever and ever, Amen."

"Amen."

She tiptoed to the front of the plane to awaken the crew. They'd learned to catch some shut eye every opportunity they could. The erratic layovers left them with a perpetual hangover like jet lag.

"We've got company."

The sound of machine gun fire lit up the night sky. The jeeps roared toward the end of the runway.

"Power up!" demanded the pilot as he scanned the controls, and began to flip a few switches.

The bright headlights lit up the long runway. They still a glimmer of hope he calculated as he hurriedly fired up the engines and quickly set a course due north. The mighty MD DC 10 began to gain speed while the welcoming barreled down the dusty dirt clearing. The guerillas had every intent-ion of grounding the plane. Then pick the fuselage apart piece by piece, bolt by bolt, like a venturesome capitalist vulture and sell it all for scrap. What treasure lay inside, they could not begin to imagine. The pilot had to insure the immunity of the contents at all costs. Better to go out in a blaze of glory, a fiery inferno and consume everything and one aboard rather than give up the deadly cargo into enemy hands.

The opposing forces, one metal behemoth and a rag tag wrangler rustling rebels were about to clash, head to head.

The guerillas unleashed a firestorm of gunfire at the ground beneath the midsection of the DC 10. The most stable albeit delicately outfitted part of the airplane. Site of the surgical suite, microscopes and countless prepared Ebola slides. And one contaminated container He had an idea.

"Hold the fort!" he commanded his copilot.

He made his way through the romper room. Ere it could erupt into a ruckus, he deployed the screen and projector to distract the kids woken by all the commotion. An old rerun, a Bugs Bunny, and

Quick Draw McGraw and his side kick Baba Looey blazing saddles type western cartoon.

The interior of the aircraft now acclimatized to the fierce gun slinging outside near the border between Zambia and Mozambique.

The gunmen blew several of the tires of the DC 10 out and almost upon them. The final confront-ation imminent.

"I can't hold her!" yelled the pilot about to cut a swath through the jungle. He had to get the bird into the air.

The jeeps roared under the fuselage then hurriedly pulled simultaneous u turns and hauled ass in a futile attempt to catch the plane. The captain reached for the cap of the canister. He quickly unscrewed it. The jiggling of the plane caused some of the contents to splash onto his forearm. He knew he was screwed. He lit a handkerchief doused in anesthetic from a lidocaine syringe stuffed into the canister and opened the emergency exit. He hurled the flaming piñata at the crazed killers. It was the next best thing in lieu of evasive maneuvers or expelling shrapnel at ensuing enemy missile or man pad attacks. The container spun topsy-turvy end over end like a satellite returning to earth on final reentry and burnout.

"Gotcha!" shouted the ring leader. The guerillas loaded the shoulder mounted rocket propelled grenade and found the target.

"Bull's eye!" shouted the captain jubilantly as the heat seeking trailblazer struck the canister. It burst into a brilliant fireball narrowly missing the aircraft and killed two birds with one stone - the deadly Ebola extract and enemy missile attack. The kids watched the fireworks outside intently, curiously with both confusion and elation, immensely grateful to have regained their sight. The DC 10 sustained minor damage by the blast as it soared into the night sky. The pilot passed the kids enthralled by the cartoons and what they thought were staged performances outside. Spared the short end of the fuse to an even shorter life, their eager innocent minds in time would learn just how lucky they truly were.

"If there's one thing I can't stand, it's being grounded" chuckled the copilot still in shock. The blazing inferno like a roaring campfire from a remote safari soon faded from sight.

"You earned your wings today. I'm proud of you." The pilot resumed command. He set a course due east toward the rising sun on the distant horizon and in an attempt to distance himself from the dark continent forever if he could. The only reminder, an itching burning scar on his forearm that slowly insidiously clawed its way into the subdermal layers of his skin. They veered from their usual flight path to figure out how they'd continue their ever growing treacherous call of duty.

"Come in over. Come in Air Mad, Come in. Is anyone out there?" asked Barry as he dejectedly tossed the microphone onto the dashboard of the boat.

"Looks like we're on our own."

"The Ebola outbreak and quarantine must be far worse than anyone expected."

"They always leave a few military frequencies open." Bernie tried to tap into secure channels frequented by only USAMRIID and a few emergency networks.

"This is Orbis One. Over."

"In the wink of an eye."

"Who is this?"

"The last resort." The nervous voice seemed sane enough.

The pilots looked at each other rather puzzled. The weak signal came from a remote rock in the Indian Ocean. The pilots instantly regained their bearings. The site of many a well deserved layover they recalled with such fond memories.

"Reset a course ENE for Victoria. Let's get this party started" quipped the seasoned chief pilot.

"Yes!" came a jubilant reply in the wee hours of the morning. Likely a few clubbers on an all night bender mused the crew. "The darkest hour is always right before the dawn."

The civilized savages sighed in relief. Their prayers might've been answered.

"I knew we'd find a way off this rock, come out smelling like a rose in fact"…said Emma referring to the Catharanthus Roseus.

The precious cargo fit snugly in their backpack Small and inconsequential to the naked eye, but could it pack a punch. 264 of the vials, 4 years of blood, sweat and tears rolled into the experimental vaccine that could potentially save millions of lives

lay on the edge of the countertop covered in bottles of rum, coconut juice….The most unlikely of places for the source of the concoction to end the spread of pain and suffering of Ebola and various forms of cancer.

"God oft chooses the most miserable wretches. His grace knows no boundaries, no limits" reflected the resilient scientists. "Add never say never , do or die. Let's call a spade a spade."

"We've shoveled a lot of shit, peeled a few petals in our lives ere we found the real treasure staring us squarely in the eyes, right in front of us."

Emma blushed, a slightly brighter red than the ink petals. She peeled a few off.

"He loves me" turning to Bernie. "He loves me" turning toward Barry. "He loves me not…" She was torn asunder by the last petal. "He loves me." She looked up at the pair of brilliant albeit uncon-ventional cads. Like irresistible loving puppy dogs.

She'd leave the impossible decision to the very end.

The unscheduled landing startled the small control tower on Mahe. Their immediate concern was a military coupe, during the quarantine, or Air Mad, to capture pillage and plunder all the exports destined for the mainland.

"This is Orbis. Requesting clearance on final approach. " The massive MD DC 10 seemed to wink at several UAV's, property of the Seychelles Public Defense Force and US Army. Obnoxiously buzzing about like a swarm of RC toys as it neared the end of the tarmac.

"You got it."

"Where were the drones when we needed them?" asked the copilot pissed off by the lack of air support.

"Might have to borrow a couple MQ-Reapers when we cross the continent on the rebound."

"Nothing like the sound of friendly fire when you need it."

The passengers' eyes were wide open, receptive to the novel experiences growing by leaps and bounds every day. Destined to make a full, speedy recovery with the newer vaccines.

The tiny tots were whisked along the Victoria-Providence highway to a waiting infirmary for further observation. Divine providence certainly played a part in their miraculous heroic rescue, desperate departure and bumpy ride to safety.

9: The Eyes Have It

> "The voyage of discovery
> is not in seeking new land-
> scapes but in having new
> eyes."
>
> - Marcel Proust, author
> "In Search of Lost Time"

The large round illuminous orbs like giant alien eyes beamed down onto center stage in the main lab deep inside the RV Neil Armstrong. The team slowly slid the massive slimy cartilaginous carcass onto the long shiny stainless steel table, then delicately sliced the large dorsal fin off.

"Fetch a pretty penny in some parts. Coveted since the Ming dynasty, prized for boosting sexual potency, preventing heart disease…." said Dr Hatfield.

"Yet, no preventative cancer properties what soever" noted Charlie. "Cartilage is avascular."

"Let's see what we've got" suggested Dr Hatfield like a child about to peer into a cereal box in quest of the elusive prize at the bottom.

A series of long leather straps laboriously rolled the massive beast onto it's dorsal surface exposing it's great white belly and a conical row of razor sharp teeth. Fleshy sinewy strands hung from the corners of it's mouth.

"Let 'er rip."

The giant serrated teeth of the jigsaw punctured the proboscis at the juncture of the lower jaw just above the s shaped heart. The jigsaw quickly unzipped the beast, nearly 21 feet in length.

She split open and spilled the bloody decomposing contents onto the shiny surface. An entire upper torso, arms, head and shoulders above the lower disemboweled half. Several Egyptian vultures still latched onto the irresistible fleshy fiesta resistance spewed out onto the table.

"Phewww." Charlie leaned over the edge of the table. She could not contain the queasy feeling in her gut then quickly grabbed and lifted her mask over her head before hurling her lunch.

"Bingo." Dr Hatfield was elated with the catch of the day. A veritable three ring circus certain to give them more clues about the nature of the naval tragedy.

Charlie rose from her hunched position. The stone cold killer's eyes seemed to follow her every move. She walked around to the other side and made a startling discovery.

"Huh? an albino…wait a minute."

Surprised to find the shark exhibited the same feature as many of the other victims. Distinct multicolored eyes.

"What do you make of this doc?" Dr Hatfield was beside himself.

"What are the chances that our old friend here has not only been exposed to the ebola virus, albeit his cartilaginous structure practically precludes him from harboring the virus. A poor host indeed. The chances of ebola completely foreign to their ecosystem, residing in his eye are slim to remote."

"You mean he may be harboring an 'illegal alien'?"

"Let's find out." The virologist made a slow cross corneal incision then aspirated the contents of the dull lifeless eye into the ship's vacu flow.

The relatively clear liquid like potent tropical punch in a blender awaited only the push of a button.

"Chris…"

"I'm on it." The resident extracted the essence of the eyeball and quickly prepared the specimen on a slide.

"If the resilient virus like some of the omega 3 fatty acid producing bacteria we've found at extreme depths and pressures were to 'spread it's wings' so to speak…." stated Dr Hatfield forebodingly as he grabbed the scavenger vulture by the neck. He tossed the brownish head, the result of eating feces whenever the opportunity arose, like a diaper onto the adjacent stainless steel dissection table.

"It's not airborne yet, is it?"

"No, I don't believe so, not in the traditional sense." But they'd soon uncover a big piece of the puzzle he sensed. His hands shook. Inspite of the best double gloving precautions, he couldn't force himself to make the first cut.

"You know you're nearing retirement when..." quipped Charlie. "Here, let me do the honors" as she relinquished his grip on the scalpel.

"I don't know what came over me." He felt a chill, then a shiver rush up and down his spine. He lifted his visor. The room became blurry...He hit his head on the edge of the unforgiving stainless steel and fell to the floor. Half his face was bathed in the bloody infected effluent. The poison quickly found the corner of his mouth as if by design.

Charlie quickly bent down and raised his head from what she felt could only be a certain death sentence. Not quick either. Slow, insidious, painful. Waiting while all the cells of his body liquefied and fell apart.

"I'm falling for you" he quipped, his sense of humor likely to accompany him to an early premature burial. Scratch that, cremation.

"I've got you. You….?!" She peered nervously into his eyes. They both knew what was in store. It was a race against the clock to come up with a couple of answers. Share them with the world. "Start spreadin' the news" before the menace became airborne again. "It's us or it!"

"Why? Why him?" she said as she slumped against the wall of the shower. Her mentor, his brilliant mind. His brash and brazen bravado is what she'd miss the most. His ornery, odd way of seeing the world. The mad hatter had met his match.

“Damn it. This is definitely not the end!” she declared, determined to give him a few more years “In fact it’s just the beginning.” The irrefutable evidence, a death sentence lay at the other end of the long shiny metal eyepiece of her scanning electron microscope. Ebola’s signature, the shepherd’s crook, the characteristic unmistakable u – turn, the ‘9’.

“By hook or by crook, by God!” she declared.

The discovery, not only the first of it’s kind, but the conclusive causal link of a clearly defined species to species transmission. The inevitable airborne spread of the disease, not in the conventional sense, confirmed. The unbelievable resilience of Ebola to mutate indefinitely, reside in any host, in any environment. By land, sea or air. “Heck it’s likely an extremophile not even from here” she said out of the blue.

"You might be onto something" said Dr Hatfield from under his multi layered malaria tent like impermeable plastic netting." The break-through is what he needed to redeem himself. His tarnished legacy, thanks to all the ill wishing fools. The professional quacks and charlatans persecuting him. The malicious lawyers and legal system forever taunting him, tearing him down, defaming, libeling, slandering. In the end it was a tiny yet formidable foe that destiny had sent to seal his fate. More powerful than any of his two legged adver-saries. A fitting, final curtain call he felt. And he was the one that made the historical discovery. His name would live on in infamy, in scientific jour-nals, textbooks, just like the man who first set foot on the moon. The very name inscribed on the side of the vessel, that is if and only if mankind were to survive. "By God! We have to let the world know!"

"I hear yuh" concurred Charlie and the rest of the team standing by his bedside.

The vessel was midway between the shores of the new world and the old ,in the most treacherous stretch of the Atlantic past the Flemish Cap …no man's land for many fishing expeditions. Like the ill fated Apollo 13 mission which merely passed by the earth's only satellite, yet found a way to return safely to earth. The RV Neil Armstrong had to get back to the American mainland to share the data, step up the production of viable vaccines by the boatload, synthesize any and all experimental clinical trials before it was too late.

His words, like Armstrong's declaring man's never ending quest for new horizons and worlds to explore. Well a significant small step, hell a giant leap was made to insure we'd still have a viable inhabitable home to come back to.

The wide eyed team lapped it all up like a sacred sermon on the mount. Their mission as clear as the swirling eddies in the Erlenmeyer flasks, bulbous glassware and assorted paraphernalia that filled the decks of discovery. They began to test every vaccine at their disposal. The countless concoctions even the military had coughed up back in Casablanca. They had a fighting chance now that they knew 'the eyes have it'. No matter what avian, land based animal or sea species.

The aircrew swirled the last of their enticing elixirs and washed down the tantalizing sea food treats that their civilized savage hosts had procured.

"One more for the road" quipped the captain as he perused the flight plan quickly penciled on the large Mercator map.

"It'll be touch and go from here on in. I can't promise you anything" he said as his finger did the walking over no man's land, Somalia and the treacherous pirate infested waters. Countless sea merchants had been taken hostage demanding outrageous out of this world ransoms in the hundreds of millions. The pirates like keen shrewd businessmen fueled many more terrorist startups and training camps on the Arabian peninsula.

"Nothing but blue skies. Smooth sailing from here on in" boasted Barry prematurely. "We'll have the best air support, thanks to the good ole US AF. A couple F135 Lightning II's on routine training maneuvers from Diego Garcia in the Indian Ocean and a fleet of MQ 9 Reaper drones."

"That's the easy part. Presuming we make landfall. After that, it's a whole other ball game."

He pointed to the empty wasteland from one coast to the other across the vast continent. If we evade enemy fire in the mountainous regions of Ethiopia, we must cross the Sudan and then ….the Sahara. The pilot drew a dotted line in the sand bordering Chad, Libya, Niger then bisected Algeria ere he marked off the coastline of Morocco up into Gibraltar.

"I place our chances at 50:50."

"That's a helluva lot better than a big goose egg."

"You've made several crossings across Africa before."

"But this. This is a game changer" referring to the countless children crippled even blinded by the emerging viral threat.

"So's this!" stated Bernie. "He patted the padded briefcase. "Our magic bullets."

The pilots demeanor perked up. Dr Gum had piqued their interests and hopes.

"Don't look at me. It's something the boys have been cooking up back in the jungle…" said Emma.

The pilots eyed them suspiciously.

"You want us to smuggle drugs or contraband? This is a purely humanitarian mission."

"She means Madagascar. An American funded university cancer research lab. Completely legit."

"We stumbled onto something. Able to kill two birds with one stone you might say."

"No shit?" They found the far fetched story hard to believe. "Piled higher and deeper than the dodo doodoo in the harbor."

"Come on."

"It's true. The concoction , CEV7 is it? It saved my life. I swear" said Emma in their defense as a desperate move, their last resort.

"I'll buy it. What have we got to lose?" he said facetiously laughing nervously.

The MD DC 10 was given final clearance to depart.

"Good luck!" wished Seychelles ATC. "And God speed."

"Luck's a very thin wire between survival and disaster, and not many people can keep their balance on it" said the copilot. Hunter Thompson's immortal words had set the tone for the entire trip.

"I feel like the first lady on Airforce One" declared Emma on likely the last leg of her whirlwind round the world globetrotting good will tour.

Accompanied by a strong visible deterrent force; The pilots in the ever battle ready F 35 Lightning

IIs gave the thumbs up then bolted down the run-way in a fiery blaze of glory. The small posse of MQ 9 predator drones were soon aloft to ride side saddle.

"Victoria, we're a go."

As if bidding adieu to a former reigning monarch, the fate of the free world once again hung in the balance. Only a few freedom fighters to lead the resistance, the charge of a light, bright, never say never brigade brought together by fate?

Divine intervention? What have you, but so be it, there you have it. They were bolting toward the coastline like the flyboys bearing down on Tokyo during the 'Doolittle Raid', the first surprise attack on the Japanese homeland on April 18, 1942 following the fateful day of infamy Dec 7, 1941.

They had so much to do, yet so little time.

The large eye inscribed on the side of the flying hospital was soon caught in the cross hairs of the gunsights of a band of beady eyed Somali pirates out on a scouting party. They wiped their sweaty brows then refocused. The eye in the sky was staring back them as if to stare them down. They flew into a fit of rage, more determined than ever to bring them down to their level and make them beg for mercy.

"Allah akbar" they shouted as they shoved the projectile into the long tube. The gentle tossing of the waves impaired their aim. Their misguided ways and means meant Orbis, the big bird leading the smaller flock might have a fighting chance.

A plume of smoke and a distinct heat signature was instantly picked up in the F35's pilot's helmet display system, an elaborate array of sensors like in the glass cockpit.

"We've got a live one!" said the composed pilot as he zoomed in on the target. A small discretely disguised fishing trawler off the shores of Mogadishu. The pirates had likely pirated the training videos made by Mogadishu rebels during the infamous US Army raid in 1993. The footage allegedly served as a 'how to' bring down a Black Hawk helicopter training video for Sadam Hussein's regime.

"Roger that" concurred his wing mate.

The erratic rapidly rising trail of smoke was instantly on the Orbis' tail on a direct intercept trajectory.

"They're firing at us!" shouted Emma from the classroom. Her eagle eyes spotted the distinct cloud out of the corner of her eye. The pilots took evasive action and veered the plane to port and prayed..

It was over in an instant. Locked and loaded, the trawler was easy pickens for the fighter pilots. “Let’s let ‘em eat crow!” quipped one of the navy’s finest.

The F 35’s sounded the trumpets, then struck like lightning…. They rained down fire and ‘Brimstone’, the deadly evolution of the hellfire ‘fire and forget’ laser guided supersonic missiles (450m/s) It found the elusive targets in an instant. The MQ 9 ‘grim’ reapers AGM 114 hell-fire missiles added insult to injury with several spot on strikes. The trawler was torn in two in a thunderous explosion and sent the Somali rebels into the air like fireworks on the 4th of July.

“Woohoo!”

"US one, pirates zero" stated the scorekeeper. Bernie kept his eyes peeled for any more nefarious activity as the plane approached the arid rugged coastline near the Horn of Africa marked by color-ful coral reefs, dotted with newly developed

resorts.

"You're on your own" stated the F35 pilot, then rapidly veered off to comb the Gulf of Aden and scope out the 'blessed isle' of Socotra off the Horn.

"Good luck and God speed." The pilots then repeatedly rolled their wings as if to wave good bye then roared off. The Reaper drones maintained a presence all the way up to the tip of Somalia ever ready for any peculiar pirate plot. "Trouble's always a brewin' round the bend."

More pirates surged to the spot to fill the hiatus left by their predecessors like the never ending tidal action of the Indian Ocean.

"Landing gear light's giving me a headache. The warning lights have come on sporadically ever since the mad dash from Zambia."

"Roger that."

The flying eye pilots corrected their course setting heading for Addis Ababa for an unscheduled 'pit stop.' They were denied access in light of the Ebola outbreak. It had already spread and ravaged the coastal cities along the Red Sea.

"AXU" stated the knowledgeable aviator.

"Excuse me" said Barry as he stepped into the cockpit curiously inspecting the maze of screens, instruments and buttons.

"An audio engineer's paradise" he quipped.

"Radio gaga" snapped the pissed off pilot.

"Pick-ing a receptive crowd and landing spot is getting harder and harder these days inspite of our rock star status" he replied.

"Definitely long enough. Some 7874 ft.

"Didn't they deliver the Axum Obelisk in an Antonov 124 there in '05?"

"Yeah. They did. AXU it is."

They veered starboard heading due north.

The tall inscribed granite stele, an odd marker for an underground burial chamber indeed. It paled in comparison to the true treasure that awaited their eyes and a fortunate few only.

Emma anxiously awaited the unexpected detour. Her fiancé had oft told her tall tales of a cherished Christian artifact housed in a chapel there. The mere mention of the word 'chapel' had sent her spirits soaring. The touch down proved touch and go. The DC 10 barely limped to the end of the asphalt runway. Its wheels wobbled having sustained serious damage during the rebel raid.

"Made it on a wing and a prayer."

"I'm afraid you might be grounded for some time" stated the Axum mechanic. African aviation maintenance records were abysmal at best. 10 times the number of crashes and incident reports. Spare parts hard to come by.

"No can do!" said Bernie defiantly. "We need to get emergency medical supplies to Morocco Stat."

The mechanic's eyes lit up.

"Perhaps a profitable exchange can be arranged."

"This is no time for trivial pursuits" snapped Bernie. "Lives are at stake."

"Millions" added Barry.

"Morocco? Casablanca, Bogey's bar, no?"

"No. I mean yes. We'll take you there. If and only if you get big bird here off the ground ASAP! capiche?"

He nodded eagerly.

"Is there anything we can do? To give you a hand?"

"Why don't you pray that I find the…parts you need… over there."

The mechanic pointed to a wanted type poster depicting the Chapel of the Tablet.

"It's the chapel!" said Emma astonished.

"Let's get her to the church on time. And you, you get us to Casablanca on time!"

"Guarded by a blind priest, the only man allowed to 'look' at the coveted artifact in the Chapel of the Tablet, the original Ark of the Covenant."

"You don't say? The Ark? The tablets, the ten commandments etched in stone by the very finger of God?"

"Divine 'heat' from the Tablets had allegedly cracked the stones in the inner sanctum. That's why it was rebuilt and moved here. A new guardian is chosen ere the death of the predecessor. He carries on the tradition, stationed there until his death, and so on."

"What a horrible way to waste away in nowhereville" said Barry sadly. "Dumb blind luck."

"Keeper of the faith. Faithful and true to the very bitter end."

They ruminated over the history and irrefutable fate of mankind.

"If only we'd read the top 10 list, let alone the maintenance manual for mankind. We'd be miles ahead."

"Free will, huh? Where did that get us?"

"Into the mess we're now in. A pretty pickle."

"Call someplace paradise...kiss it goodbye. In time even the Seychelles will be overrun by the Ebola pandemic in its relentless march round the globe like all the other rulers, Genghis Khan, Ming, Alexander the Great, Caeser, Napolean, Hitler...., It's only a matter of time."

They patted the absorbent Axum sponge on the shoulder, sitting silently on his perch outside the sanctum. The blind guardian was in a way, perhaps better off, spared from witnessing the wrath and scourge of the disease destined to mark the end of the world.

"May you find good fortune. Peace be with you my brothers and sisters" he said ere they left. The little black Buddha seemed to wink at them then sensed an evil presence nearby.

"You're in good hands. You have to hurry." he said in a soft spoken voice then stared skyward.

10: Land’s End

> “Man cannot discover new
> oceans until he has the courage
> to lose sight of the shore.”

- Andre Gide, author, Nobel
  Prize winner in Literature in
  1947

The RV Neil Armstrong, USNS Comfort and Mercy set their headings toward the new land. Their destination, unknown like the former venturesome flotilla of three small trading vessels the Nina, Pinta and Santa Maria, designed merely to roam the Mediterranean. They had far surpassed the expectations and limits imposed by the flat earth followers and narrow minded scientific community of their day. To boldly go where no man had gone before, where only eagles dare as the US president had so succinctly stated. The eastern extremity of the United States just beyond the horizon. The majestic rugged coastline of Cape

Cod, Massachusetts within reach. They'd find the fork in the road, soon. Forced to go north to the most modern facilities at Mass General or divert south along Long Island, Rhode Island, Connecticut and beeline for the newest medical breakthroughs awaiting them at NYU, Sunnybrook etc. The Brooklyn Bridge, Ellis Island and the all too familiar Lady Liberty beckoning countless lost souls before them were not even so much as a thought in the minds of the natives. Manhattan, bartered from the Canarsee Indians by the Dutch, whose fur trade presence on Governor's Island expanded for about 60 guilder, or $24. No one could've foreseen the era of prosperity and rise to the pinnacle of global prominence. Wall street, venture capitalism at it's finest. Trillions in misguided hedge funds, retirement portfolios, junk bonds and annuities. It may not be worth a plugged nickel soon as the imminent hostile takeover by an unwanted pesky little start up entity loomed. Sordid rumors circulated and soon spread rampantly. The mere mention of the name ebola struck fear and widespread panic into the hearts of the boardrooms, amongst the stock traders in ALL global markets. The brightest and best minds could not begin to calculate the economic costs nor ramifications if the virus gained a beach head at Battery Park and cut across the trading floors at the NYSE. Would they witness the ultimate demise and collapse of the American empire? A swan

song, a final curtain call?

Port authorities were pressured by the powers that be all the way up the food chain to the mayor, governors, even the State legislature passed legislation to impede the passage of the infected vessels.

"I see" said the captain of the Comfort as he charted the rough waters off the Cape. The sister ship Mercy was shown nothing of the sort of compassion and warm embrace generations of immigrants were shown. The stakes were too high. The Ebola virus had run its course ravaging all aboard. He knew they'd likely repel any naval 'invasion' and scuttle her off Martha's Vineyard or Woods Hole. Just another diving attraction.

He was torn. In dire straits. He'd soon have to make a dramatic decision. Facing a similar futile situation as the commander of the Mystique of the Seas, he feared the end was near.

Deck upon deck had turned to sealed steel stacked sarcophagi. The victims entombed and preserved inside the catacombs of the floating mausoleum. The experimental vaccines could not contain the insatiable contagion. The dead were simply shut off from the rest of the ship. Water tight doors sealed their fate like the lost souls trapped in the boiler rooms and below the waterline in the lower decks aboard the 'unsinkable' Titanic.

The option to flood the entire lot in naval fuel or av gas and light her up like a roman candle was not an option he stated defiantly. The mounting press-ure to prevent a pandemic from spreading across

the tristate harbor mow paramount.

"He had no choice but to soon abandon ship as he shot several rounds of flares into the air. Like bombs bursting in air on the 4th of July, the distress signal was seen for miles off shore. Mistaken as a celebration of sorts. The captain counted down the hours and minutes. He'd soon be faced with an awful decision. He'd either be forced to stay adrift at sea indefinitely… a veritable virus ridden vessel waiting to be ravaged, pillaged and plundered by teams of hazmat and medical professionals, a gruesome ghost ship or be forced to ground and scuttle her on the rocky shoals off Cape Cod or Long Island. Either way he'd go out in a blaze of glory.

"Sir what shall I tell them?" stated a seaman frantically. He'd trudged through the bloody sludge of human remains likely infected himself. The captain saw the whites or rather multicolored corneas of his blood shot eyes.

"The night is always darkest before the dawn." Neither a very religious man, he sought refuge in a passage from Matthew 6:34 KJV.

"Take therefore no thought for the morrow, for the morrow shall take thought for the things of itself. Sufficient unto the day is the evil thereof."

He knew the cadet would not last the night.

"Thank you, sir." He disappeared into dark foreboding catacombs of the ship with what little comfort the captain of the hospital ship, a massive converted supertanker, could provide.

In the sick bay of the Neil Armstrong, a group of dedicated scientists gathered by Dr Hatfield's bedside. His faithful Tilly cap hung on an oxygen tank never far from his side. His dying wish was to bury him with his signature trademark. He was on his last legs,

"What would I have done without you? All of you. He peered at them from his bleary bloodshot eyes, dripping from even his ear canals…the seasoned scientist looked like a gaunt, grim doppelganger of his former self. He'd cried a river of… blood by the looks of the soaked red sheets under the plastic tent pumped with pressurized oxyen, which only fueled the feisty inhabitant's advance faster and more furiously. Dr Hatfield knew he'd soon pay the pied piper his last respects ere he'd lead him off into the promised land.

"So close yet so far."

"Come on lad. Spit it out."

"We're only a fortnight from the Cape. All of Wood's Hole is waiting to welcome us back."

"You're a hero just like Armstrong."

"Good. It'll be good to get back home."

He slipped into a comatose state. The meds and a private stash of fortified hybridized canna-bidiol marijuana had stopped the seizures.

"Let him rest."

Charlie led the despondent researchers back to their posts. The situation seemed dire. Death knocking on their doorstep. She peered out of the starboard porthole and could only imagine the mayhem magnified a thousand fold aboard the Mercy.

"Have mercy on their souls" she prayed.

They paid their last respects and departed from the tiny garden next to the chapel. The procession of pilots and pioneering scientists left on a somber note ready to tackle the last treacherous leg on their mission. The blind priest urged them to leave im-mediately. He sensed the proximity of the rebels.

They spotted the Axum aviation mechanic swing at least three times ere he tossed the large wrench onto the bench.

“Don’t ask.”

“Don’t tell. I don’t want to know” stated the pilot.

“You’re good. Yeah. Good to go” he stated proud of his accomplishment.

“All she needed was a minor adjustment.”

He packed prepared for the long road to hoe through the Sahara ahead of them.

“Well then let’s shove off” declared the pilot somewhat skeptically.

“NOW!” he shouted as a barrage of obnoxious rebels guns a blazing came out the scrub brush to ambush the Flying Hospital. Obviously perturbed by the only trusted mechanic’s exodus out of Ethiopia.

“Here we go again!” said Barry as he bolted up the stairs.

The Orbis barreled down the long asphalt strip. The enraged Ethiopians, intent on preventing a 'brain drain', expressed their opinion in a direct way. Rounds of ammo ricocheted off the tarmac. Several found the aluminum fuselage, tearing gaping holes in the outer shell. A few stray rounds clipped the cockpit. The shrapnel grazed the copilot's right arm. A steady drip fell onto the console about to burst into flames as a result of a short circuit at any second.

The tired team clutched the chairs of the class-room seats confident in the power of prayer, the short sermon led by one blind guardian. They were airborne before you could say Haile Selassie.

"Dumb blind luck!"

The aircraft soared across the Sudan border… It's tail feathers ruffled, and it's landing gear jam-med.

"Ahhh? What did I tell you, she's as good as new" rejoiced the jaunty jalopy man of all trades.

The pilot spared them the 'good news' until later. Par for the course as African aviation maintenance went.

"Yeah, good as new." He turned to the copilot. They were smooth sailing. The problem lay in the next layover in Gibraltar. How could they conceivably land the big bird?

The lush banks of the Nile, a tropical oasis bordering no man's land to either side of Khartoum were the last signs of life and civilization light years away. They'd soon transcend time and space upon entering the barren endless sandy wasteland and scorching heat waves.

"Hang onto your shorts." Neither short nor

sweet, beads of sweat began to fall from the brows of all aboard. The rounds of ammo or the mechanic may have inadvertently switched a few key relays or used substandard parts for the air conditioning conked out. Their worst fear, a fire onboard. He perished the thought of ditching near Lake Chad, a reliable runway in a pinch. Considering the vital water supply serving some 70 million people throughout Niger, Chad, Nigeria and Cameroon was reduced by 95%. Steadily shrinking for decades, the endless salt flats dotted in islands provided little relief for the pilot. He had no choice but to deliver the precious, priceless CEV7 vaccine on time. He trusted the former Fedex airframe implicitly. It was all the meddling fools that tinkered with it he could not.

"This is gonna get bumpy" as they approached the mountain range, hydraulic and fuel line levels suddenly dropped.

"We took a hard hit at Axum."

"We can't get a God damned break!" blared the pilot, One of the engines burst into flames. An act of God is not on the agenda, not mow!" he yelled defiantly. His patience worn thin yet quickly extinguished it. The DC 10 dared not lose another drop of the hybrid aviation biofuel or a touchdown in Gibraltar would be out of the question let alone reach the American mainland.

The specialists had little time to reflect on their sordid shenanigans and life changing experiences yet they decided to give it a go. Fearing they'd soon fall from the sky in a fiery fireball and have their ashes strewn all over some God forsaken sector of the Sahara they decided to share their sordid stories. Up to now, their mundane, inconsequential lives were never put to a real test.

"Truth or dare" suggested Barry. They faced one another perhaps for the last time. "A good a time as any to spill the beans." not only to relinquish any deep dark secrets they may have harbored since their early college days but share some insights, a strand of hope to hang onto.

"I'll go first" said Emma. "I want to thank you all from the bottom of my heart. Without you, I wouldn't be here. Swear to God, cross my heart hope to...."

"Yeah yeah" said Barry, "Enough doom and gloom. You're welcome. This isn't an Academy Award acceptance speech. Nothing scripted, just call it like it is, straight from the heart, off the top of your head, off the cuff."

The pilot overheard the honest admissions.

"When I get back, if there's anything to go back to, I will take that extra week coming to me. Heck

I will retire! Settle on some remote rock. My first mate, my girl Friday by my side, every day of the week."

"What about you Emma? What are your plans?"

"I was lost, but now I'm found. If a wretch like me is given a second chance…I won't waste another second, second guessing myself. My fiancé God rest his soul, did open my eyes. I'll probably volunteer for some humanitarian organization."

"I've given too much of my free time to charity, all these years. Gratis. They can't afford me.."

"What did it ever get you? Was it worth it?"

"All the lives saved. The look of gratitude in their eyes to be given a new lease on life…. Priceless.

"Regrets?"

"I have a few" Emma said disheartened. "I didn't have a chance to have kids, see them grow up, watch them graduate from college…."

"You're still a spring chicken. Live a little. Take a chance…" Bernie encouraged her looking deeply in her eyes. "Your whole future lies ahead of you. Right in front of your eyes." The group recognized the blatantly obvious invitation.

"You're not proposing are you?"

"Not this very second. Give it a minute. You'll know where to find me" he quipped. He got up and nervously paced back and forth. The endless sea of swirling, ever shifting sand dunes on either side of the aircraft unnerved him. 3.6 million square miles.

"Go ahead. Tell her… how you feel."

"Take a leap… of faith."

He hoped no one would have to jettison or exit too prematurely.

Emma was overwhelmed. The look of love was in her eye.

"Life is what happens to you while you're busy making other plans" reiterated Barry. "The Beatles is the best you could come up with?"

"Yeah. Love is all you really need. It's too bad the rest of this wretched rock is too busy killing, blowing one another up in the name of some god? some misguided, delusional ideology. No tolerance for one another. Where is the love?"

The Black Eyed Peas lyrics popped into his head…

"You're right. There's no point in moping, mulling over what might've been."

"That's it."

" Now you're talking."

"Grab the bull by the horns. Horn of Africa excluded."

They had crossed that perilous bridge. A bridge too far from reason.

Bernie observed several mountain ranges that looked like a lunar landscape. The Atlas still a few hours away. He calibrated the compass app on his smartphone to get his bearings.

"Those are the Air Mts. of northern Niger. Nothing but African wild dogs, a little like the laughing hyena. Eat you alive."

"Ha, ha." He'd never fully grown accustomed to all the turbulence no matter how many military missions he'd flown. He got weak in the knees.

"Atta boy" said the pilot persuasively.

"You have fallen for me."

"Truth or dare" interjected Barry. "Come on yuh big chicken. Bock, bock."

"I…I . Oh what the hell. Emma will you …"

An air pocket jiggled the cabin sufficiently to send Emma plummeting into his arms. In lieu of an actual wedding band he'd resourcefully wrapped a couple pretty pink petals from a periwinkle flower around a metal ring, the seal from one of the CEV7 vials.

She recalled playing the game pulling the petals to the tune of 'he loves, me, he loves me not….' Barry appeared dejected.

"I will."

The band fit like a glove.

"It's been a long time comin'" declared Bernie. A few details and kinks needed to be worked out. Sign the divorce papers.

"Well, this is a first. Love at first sight. A couple that sees eye to eye" quipped the pilot.

He had to explain and fast.

"What I think he means is most of us never seize the opportunity, the day. Carpe diem..".

"Shut up Barry" snapped Emma.

The lucky couple peered into each other's eyes as if they'd known each other for a lifetime.

"Just don't ask us to take another leap of faith" said Bernie as the plane caught a few more air pockets. The bumpy rollercoaster ride of their lives had only just begun.

The terrain rose noticeably.

"Ladies and gentlemen please note the No Smoking signs" he said facetiously. A trail of smoke…likely the loss of hydraulic fluid made a landing virtually impossible.

"Barry, here are your parting gifts" as they shoved a couple parachutes into the virologist and mechanic's hands. "

"Every passenger gets one on AxAir" he quipped.

"Your stop's coming up Ahmed. Barry's stop is on the other side of the ...prepare for final descent." They plotted a course through the Grand Atlas Mts. of Morocco down to Casablanca.

The copilot opened an emergency exit. True to his word, the aircraft mechanic …descended to his new home. Barry prepared for his jump. The precious back pack filled with about half of the CEV7 vials.

"Enough to give 'em a fighting chance.."

"Go get 'em. God Speed!"

The plane veered to the Gibraltar International runway, literally a reclaimed swath blasted from the rock. EMS from St Bernard's hospital, taxis and military escorts were poised to pick up the scruffy specialist now more important than all other dignitaries combined.

"Catch you later alligator" he signed off and stepped out into the wild blue yonder. "Be good to each other."

"Bye Barry." Emma gave him a tiny peck on the cheek. Barry touched down like a Flying Elvis, a flare in each hand... He rolled like a tumbling dice onto the tarmac. The welcoming committee whisked him into the waiting hummer like the rock star that he was.

The vital vaccines were dispersed in the ER's of St. Bernard's and synthesized as fast as they conceivably could.

"The eyes have it" declared the epidemiologist optimistically. They'd have to wait and see. CEV7 may gain the nickname VE, a victory in Europe as precious now as it was over half a century ago.

11: Providence

"We failed but in the good providence
of God apparent failure oft receives a blessing."

- Robert E. Lee, commander
Confederate Army during
The American Civil War

Orbis once again winked to an appreciative audience assembled on the runway.

"A standing ovation no less" clapped Emma.

The copilot's lifeless body slumped over the steering column.

"Mike?"

Bernie rushed into the cockpit to take his pulse both on the carotid artery on the side of his neck and his wrist to be certain.

"He's had a heart attack." Bernie eased him from the steering column. Shocked to see the bloody drops dripping from his chin. His bloodshot eyes a cause of considerable concern.

"Mike! Stay with me!"

"You won't give us a break, will you?" snapped Emma angrily as she looked out and up ahead into the Atlantic then pounded the steering column.

"We're on the home stretch" stated the seasoned pilot weakly as he activated the auto pilot and set a heading for JFK International. "You're gonna have to bring her in on your own."

"Who me?"

"Piece of cake. I'll call the shots. Time to grab the bull by the horns."

"I need a few more red bulls" he said nervously. "Haven't you heard it gives you wings."

"Calm down. It's gonna be alright. I believe in you" said Emma as she helped Bernie carry the infected pilot from the cockpit to a classroom and seated him in a upright position

Bernie withdrew a vial from the padded compart-ment and aspirated a syringe.

"It's now or never." He depressed the syringe. The coveted concoction penetrated Mike's forearm skin. The solution surged via his venous return system to the heart. From there it permeated all the cells of his body and began to work it's magic.

"Let's hope all that US grant money went to good use!"

They returned to the cockpit to assess the array of screens, controls and dials… The artificial horizon still sat squarely level.

"That's a good thing" stated Bernie slowly osmosing the dizzying data displays. "Course heading due west along the 41st parallel. 41 degrees, 23 minutes, 35 seconds."

"What does that mean?"

"If we're lucky we'll cruise right into NYC."

"How will we land?"

"I haven't figured that part out yet."

--

Three vessels Comfort, Mercy and Neil Arm-strong rapidly approached the outer extremity of the eastern seaboard. The USCG at Cape Cod immediately deployed a dynamic duo of MH-60T Jayhawk helicopters to investigate the strange signal. Marred by squelch, yet unmistakably an emergency frequency. The ever ready teams set for SAR, environmental protection and law inforcement missions dashed out to sea to get a closer look.

"Initial contact indicates a charred supertanker …precariously close to the narrow spit of land. Populated by over 370 species of birds. 80 actively breeding and nesting ere they migrate along the Atlantic seaboard up to the Arctic and as far south as Antarctica. A peculiar pattern of events had a way of creating another naval disaster. They did not need an oil tanker to wash onto the pristine pro-tected shores and spill countless gallons of crude. They were in for an even more rude awakening as they neared the vessel.

"Do you see what I see?" questioned the puzzled Coast Guard Pilot. The faint red outline of a red cross was a dead giveaway.

"Mercy Me" quipped the copilot. "I wondered what happened to the hospital ship. Carried a compliment of contaminated passengers. Ebola." They looked at one another. Dare they attempt a rescue at all if need be. They decided to hover and scour the entire three football fields of the fatally wounded and failing health by the minute. Precious seconds ticked away.

The crews of the HH 3F Pelican , the HH 3E Jolly Green Giant were the first to contact the USNS Comfort on the south side of Nantucket.

Near Long Island. They feared a similar fate had befallen the vessel. Either overrun by Ebola or all hands already lost.

"It's a dicey situation indeed. Damned if we do, damned if we don't"

"This is USCG Pelican to base. Over."

The commander peered at the large screen..

"We're in a bit of a pickle sir."

"Well spit it out."

"Can you give us an update on the Comfort and Mercy."

"Come again." An emergency red alert warning code plastered the screen. "Three vessels Comfort, Mercy and Neil Armstrong are to be detained off-shore. Under no circumstance are they permitted to land on US soil. It's a matter of National Security."

"Sir?"

RV Neil Armstrong has slipped in under the radar off Vineyard Sound not far from home. Wood's Hole inhabitants are lining up in droves for a hero's welcome.

At AFT Airport in Providence, the new corporate headquarters for Bell Helicopter Textron…the latest Bell 525 Relentless sprung into the air. An ideal photo op, the CEOs felt…Why not whisk the hero's home in the latest, most spacious fly by wire helicopter to come of age. In test flight's it performed flawlessly. Otis National Guard was alerted. The largest Aerospace Defense station in the world. Otis Airfield station directly south of the USCG station at Sandwich Gate got the green light. The only base named after a doctor, Boston General flight surgeon and pilot Jesse Otis who lost his life far too early in combat.

"A storm's a brewin'. They're essentially sitting ducks and we're Elmer Fudd, with a finger on a hair trigger to come to their rescue."

"A deadly virus of inestimable death and destructive potential gaining a foothold or beach head on American soil is unthinkable. "

To compound matters, a sighting of an erratically low flying MD DC 10 approaching the out-skirts of Martha's Vineyard unhinged them.

"Prepare to engage."

"Aye, aye sir." A squadron of F35 Lighting II's were deployed in a heartbeat. The last line of defense ere history repeated itself. The low flying behemoth squarely on a collision course with the Freedom Tower and /or lower Manhattan.

A local radio station began to broadcast on an open frequency.

“Turn it up” snapped Emma. Eager to receive a word, any sign…even from the almighty. They both recognized the Eagles ‘Last Resort’ lyrics…rather ironic and coincidental.

“Definitely a sign” concurred Emma.

They came from Providence
The one in Rhode Island
Where the old world shadows hang
Heavy in the air
She packed her hopes and dreams
like a refugee
Just as her father came across the sea
She’d heard about a place
People were smilin’
They spoke about the red man’s way
And how they loved the land
And they came from everywhere
To the Great Divide

Seeking a pace to stand

Or a place to hide….

Mike stirred and came around from all the commotion. His fever had broken and temperature subsided. He rose from his atypical chair in the front row. Startled to find himself facing the cockpit. Two foreigners at the helm? He felt queasy, far from his usual chipper self. The vaccine had dealt a knockout punch to his adversary. It was time he did the same.

"Mike? Thank God you could join us."

In his cancer /ebola therapy induced state marked by vomiting, fatigue, amnesia he didn't recognize the 'newlyweds', their honeymoon about to take a turn for the worse. In fact destined for a fatal fall. A true test of their faith in one another.

"This is Raptor Command, come in over."

Mike fumbled with the radio.

"We demand you abort your current flight path and haul your asses out of here pronto."

A deadly showdown, now imminent, seemed unavoidable.

"This is Captain Mike Connors ….." ere he completed his statement he passed out.

Emma looked at Bernie in sheer terror.

"They're gonna shoot us out of the sky!" she screamed.

Bernie responded in the nick of time.

"Alright guys. Enough's enough. We've got a vaccine aboard. To stop the spread of Ebola. It works" he said as Mike stirred groggily. "We have to land ASAP to distribute it."

"Ebola? What's he talking about? What aren't they telling us?"

"Those three ships are doomed. Guys, if we don't get these meds to them STAT, they'll all die!"

The confusing chatter was picked up by all parties concerned. Even local DJs, Good News Broadcast and radio stations all along the coast..

"Listen guys. We've got the antidote. The cure. A new vaccine that even the military doesn't know about. It's our only hope. So help me God, if you blow us out of the sky, the faces of the thousands of victims clinging on for dear life onboard those three vessels, the USNS Comfort, Mercy and RV Armstrong will be snuffed out and forever etched in your consciences!" Bernie's sermon sounded convincing.

There was a moment's silence….only the lyrics to 'Last Resort' lingered.

You can leave it all behind

Sail to Lahaina

Just like the missionaries did

So many years ago.

They even brought a neon sign,

Jesus is coming.

Brought the white man's burden down

Brought the white man's reign

Who will provide the grand design?

What is yours and what is mine?

'Cause there is no more new frontier

We have got to make it here

We satisfy our endless needs

Justify our bloody deeds

In the name of destiny

and the name of God.

Cooler heads prevailed. The aerial strike was called off.

"I can't hold her." The massive MD DC10

dropped into the middle of Martha's Vineyard ...like a bag of over ripe grapes on a deadly bombing raid. It was truly touch and go. A fatal crash could still incinerate the CEV 7 vaccine in an instant and any hope of survival.

The plane barreled in on runway 24....

The crew of Air Force One...forced to come about and take another crack at landing. The president eager to take a break from the deadly news spreading 'round the globe. Economic ruin, disease, death, and destruction triggered by an ornery insatiable little virus. Of unknown origin.

"Sir, an aircraft is jamming the runway."

"Well tell whoever it may concern that I'd like my parking space back!" quipped the President facetiously. "I'd like to throw a couple hoops."

The crew was hooped as they circled the vine-yard another time.

The plane burst into flames as it gouged it's way down the long tarmac. The first cut was the deep-est, scars that would take a long time to heal.

"Come on, let's get outta here" urged Bernie as he grabbed Emma by the waist. Her arm extended over his shoulder. Mike hung onto Bernie's other shoulder for dear life. He felt the entire weight of the world come to rest squarely on his shoulders, like the Hercules' Pillars in Gibraltar. They knelt in the smoky cockpit and hobbled out grabbing the padded briefcase. The plane reeked of a deadly concoction of avgas and hybrid biodiesel. Bernie punched the emergency exit door out. Emma

deployed the rubber raft like slide. One by one they slid from the burning DC 10. They mustered enough strength and clawed their way across the tarmac in the nick of time. The MD DC 10 burst into flames and exploded. Shrapnel was strewn across runway 24. The aircraft had not turned a blind eye. It had served fearlessly in countless humanitarian and civilian missions. Hauling everything from household goods to VCRs as a faithful Fedex frequent flyer. It saved the best for last. On it's last legs, coming home on a wing and a prayer guided by faith. Was it just dumb blind luck or divine providence? You decide.

The HH 3 E Jolly Green Giant touched down, followed by the Pelican and eventually the Bell Textron Relentless. The three weary wanderers wrapped in blankets, were escorted into the term-inal. They had definitely lost their way, but not their faith. The air crews quickly distributed the spoils, the coveted cure the civilized savages had discovered, labored tirelessly to replicate, fought tooth and nail for. The Coast Guard quickly air lifted the tiny precious cargo to the three vessels trapped in a hellish limbo in no man's land off shore.

After the flames were extinguished, the smolder-ng embers, a sad fateful reminder of what might've ended in utter tragedy, not hope.

Air Force One touched down on the Martha's Vineyard Airport. The secret service hurriedly hustled the commander in chief toward a waiting motorcade.

"Wait…just one cotton picken' minute" he stated.

"But sir…"

He stepped out of the formal procession to personally thank the three forlorn amigos ere he had to go.

The president extended a hand despite the dire warnings, misguided medical myths, ill advised secret service, all the misinformed politicians, pundits, lobbyists and journalists aboard.

"He's crazy!"

"I want to personally thank you on behalf of the American people, in fact the entire free world for your valiant acts of bravery and courage. And in the immortal words of JFK: 'We chose to go to the moon and do the other things not because they were easy but because they were hard; because those goals will serve to organize and measure the best of our energies and skills and that challenge is one we are willing to accept, one we are unwilling to postpone and one we intend to win'." He ended his longwinded sermon on a winning note.

"The true test of courage is yet to come" said

Bernie as Emma held up the makeshift

wedding

band around her ring finger. They waited with baited breath for a quick comeback

"Ha, ha. Don't lose hope! I didn't. Behind every successful man is a woman. Behind her is his wife" quipped the commander in chief erroneously quoting Groucho Marx, the other guy, usually re-served for a Presidential roast or comical cocktail conversation.

"Why don't you stop by the white house in a couple days once the smoke clears, if you're in the neighborhood. My treat."

--

Outside the Oval office in the Rose Garden a small private ceremony was in progress.

"I can't believe we're standing here."

"Like I always said 'Chance favors the

prepared mind'."

"Just a little bit of divine providence goes a long way" added Emma. The president reached for the shiny piece of polished hardware, a token of not only his gratitude, but all Americans and citizens around the world.

They took him up on his offer. They were each awarded the Congressional Gold Medal. Even Dr Hatfield made an astonishing appearance to accept his award after a miraculous recovery.

"It was touch and go. The vaccines arrived in the nick of time thanks to a brave soul of the USCG. They winched him down onto the virus riddled

deck of the vessel risking life and limb."

"Your achievements will have a lasting impact on American history and likely to be recognized long after we're gone."

Humbled by the prestigious award. They bowed, displaying their sincere heart felt gratitude.

Of course, as luck would have it, Bernie's gold medallion fell to the ground where Barney, the president's ever present Scottish terrier, snatched it from his fingertips right under his nose and dashed into the bushes. The small gathering erupted in a roar of laughter, amused by the animal's antics. There wasn't a dry eye in the house.

EPILOGUE

Some say divine intervention had a vital part to play in Will miraculously getting the vaccine to Emma. The syringe, even if perceived as a placebo had passed through countless hands like the dollar bill, the all seeing eye of God always in control? From the clandestine labs in Madagascar all the way to the Medecien Sans Frontiers on the front lines. Will sought to alleviate all the pain and suffering. Yet in an ironic twist of fate, seemingly spared the scourge of the impending global pandemic, he succumbed to the virus, as an unwary innocent carrier, yet simultaneously successfully passed the torch of discovery in the quest to eliminate the dreaded disease once and for all from the face of the earth, onto the next willing open minded group of humanitarians.

.

"And God shall wipe away all tears from their eyes; and there shall be no more death, neither sorrow, nor crying, neither shall there be any more pain: for the former things are passed away." Revelation 21:4 King James Version (KJV)

Functional lacrymal gland regeneration by transplantation of a bioengineered organ germ M.Hirayama, M.Ogawa, M. Oshima, T. Tsuji, et al.
Nature Communications Oct 1, 2013

Human lachrymal gland regeneration Perspectives and review of literature S. Tiwara, M.Javed Ali, G. Vemuganti. Saudi Journal of Opthalmology 2014 28 12-18.

Scientists regenerate fully functional tear and saliva glands. M.Ogawa, T. Tsuji. Medical News Today Oct. 5 2013.

Lacryma Christi Wine Enthusiast 2012 08 25 http://buyingguide.winemag.com/regions/italy/southern/lacrymachristivesuvio

Ebola Virus Lingers in Eyeball Even After Recovery. World News May 8, 2015. Lupkin, Sydney.

After Nearly Claiming His Life, Ebola Lurked in His Eye. NY Times May 7 2015. Grady, Denise.

Ebola Changed This Doctor's Eye Color. Popular Science. Ossala, Alexandra. May 8, 2015.
Should we diagnose rare diseases with smartphones? David Robson. Future 2014 10 17 http://www.bbc.com/future/story/20141017-the-ebola-detector-in-your-pocket

GAP Great Adventure People African Cruises
https://www.gadventures.com/trips/west-africa-cruise-cape-town-to-marrakech/XVCMDX/2015/

How many patients have been treated outside of Africa? NY Times Jan. 26, 2015
http://www.nytimes.com/interactive/2014/07/31/world/africa/ebola-virus-outbreak-qa.html?_r=0

Birds could spread Ebola CBC Dec.18, 2002
http://www.cbc.ca/news/birds-could-spread-ebola-virus-study-suggests-1.316189

Possible sexual transmission of Ebola Virus – Liberia 2015. CDC May 8, 2015. Morbidity and Mortality Weekly Report
http://www.cdc.gov/mmwr/preview/mmwrhtml/mm6417a6.htm?s_cid=mm6417a6_w

Identification of 53 Compounds that inhibit Ebola-like particle entry via repurposing screen of Approved Drugs. Emerging Microbes and Infections Dec 17, 2014
http://www.nature.com/emi/journal/v3/n12/full/emi201488a.html

Google Science Fair 2015 Grand Prize Winner - Olivia Hallisey invented an inexpensive Ebola virus field test
https://www.googlesciencefair.com/projects/en/2015/a035b3748fb27ab0f735ef30096d0cc4d15960ed3410f585c87a807c934892f4

Addendum 1st FDA approved vaccine for Ebola Virus Disease
https://www.fda.gov/news-events/press-announcements/first-fda-approved-vaccine-prevention-ebola-virus-disease-marking-critical-milestone-public-health

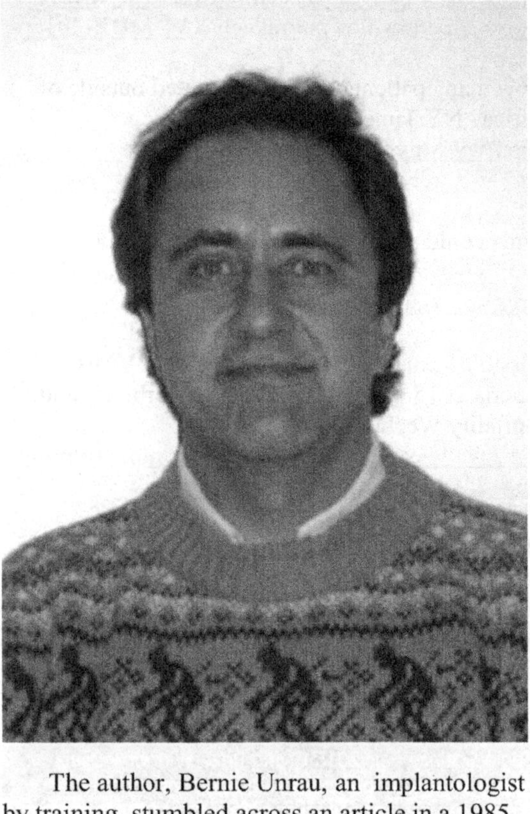

The author, Bernie Unrau, an implantologist by training, stumbled across an article in a 1985 CDA Journal entitled "Dentists as Detectives" and a four minute video back in 1989, an interview with the prolific Robin Cook, the father of the medical thriller, a physician and ophthalmologist by training, inspired Bernie to embark on a 2nd career and a new uncharted course each summer.

The central character in his novels, “Dr Gum”, a nickname he acquired from his “Gumtex” dental surgical patents which paid his way through dental and grad school. Perhaps part bumbling lieutenant Columbo or the deductive Sherlock Holmes, the imaginary detective created by Conan Doyle, also a physician/ opthalmologist. The tenacity of Dr Ryan conceived of by Tom Clancy, or the curiosity of Indiana Jones. A dash of the dapper James Bond blended, shaken and stirred into the equation the inspiration of in depth concept research of Michael Crichton and his creations or the powerful suspense of a John Grisham legalistic thriller. Or to simply bring some of his years as a dentist, implantologist, inventor and lecturer to light by engaging in espionage, elucidating an enigma, disclosing the dastardly or diabolical scheme, or dreaming up a formidable frightening future. And as the prolific Zane Grey, dentist turned novelist turned screenwriter, pen 100 books. The author has enjoyed travel, tennis, sailing, skiing, hiking, flying, reading and thinking. He is single and currently resides in Calgary, Alberta.

Books by Dr Bernie Unrau:

Terra Vista
Deadly Implant
Not A Drop
Golden Mask
Questa
Rook
Hooked
Big B
Enlightened
The Board
The ROM
New Millenium
Reflections
Submarine Slide
Sabotage
Dentinator
Ubar
Stemwinder
Pulling Strings
Meltdown
Pulpit Fiction
Confusion
Glazers
God Almighty
The Scrying
Rising
Cravings
Fantastic Voyage III
East of Aden
The X Files: The Grey Zone
Lacryma Christi

In Gold We Trust
Lion Island
Dead Hand
Dream Big
The Fifth Pillar

Screenplays by Dr Bernie Unrau:

Terra Vista
Deadly Implant
Not A Drop
Golden Mask
Questa
Rook
Hooked
Big B
Enlightened
The Board
The ROM
New Millenium
Reflections
Submarine Slide
Sabotage
Dentinator
Ubar
Stemwinder
Pulling Strings
Meltdown
Pulpit Fiction
Confusion
Glazers
God Almighty
The Scrying
Rising
Fantastic Voyage III

East of Aden
Cravings
The X Files: the Grey Zone
Chokepoint
Ultra Stealth: War Game
Phantom of the Operatory
Montauk Monster
Deep Fright
Jabberwhacky
Pandemonium
Deep Fright: Down Under
The Curse of the 7 Pagodas
Sweet Tooth
The Ice Forest
The Frozen Chosen
Insight
Subterranea
The Glass
Deep Fright: Deep Freeze
Sky Parlor
The Movie Mobile
Nightwalker
Venus' Grotto
Big Fat Liar 2
The Space Bar
Spearphish
Mind At Large
Summa Gate
Not Yet
Finger of God
Terror Island
Game Over
Salt II
Death Valley Riders
Apes & Aliens

Zombie Street
Catch Me When You Can
Bloody Mary
Raid
Bury Me Under The Volcano
The Privateers
Bond Jane Bond
You Can't Take It With You
Catch 22
The Float House
Alien Vengeance
Alien Vengeance: Raising Cain
The Great Museum Heist
Magic is in the Hare
Goldfield
Quicksilver
Bad to the Bone
In Gold We Trust
Lion Island
Dead Hand
The Fifth Pillar

Made in the USA
Monee, IL
04 November 2026

67385521R00193